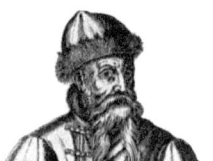

The publishing house tredition has created the series **TREDITION CLASSICS**. It contains classical literature works from over two thousand years. Most of these titles have been out of print and off the bookstore shelves for decades.

The book series is intended to preserve the cultural legacy and to promote the timeless works of classical literature. As a reader of a **TREDITION CLASSICS** book, the reader supports the mission to save many of the amazing works of world literature from oblivion.

The symbol of **TREDITION CLASSICS** is Johannes Gutenberg (1400 – 1468), the inventor of movable type printing.

With the series, tredition intends to make thousands of international literature classics available in printed format again – worldwide.

All books are available at book retailers worldwide in paperback and in hardcover. For more information please visit: www.tredition.com

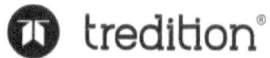

tredition was established in 2006 by Sandra Latusseck and Soenke Schulz. Based in Hamburg, Germany, tredition offers publishing solutions to authors and publishing houses, combined with worldwide distribution of printed and digital book content. tredition is uniquely positioned to enable authors and publishing houses to create books on their own terms and without conventional manufacturing risks.

For more information please visit: www.tredition.com

Hydriatic treatment of Scarlet Fever in its Different Forms

Charles Munde

Imprint

This book is part of the TREDITION CLASSICS series.

Author: Charles Munde
Cover design: toepferschumann, Berlin (Germany)

Publisher: tredition GmbH, Hamburg (Germany)
ISBN: 978-3-8491-8588-6

www.tredition.com
www.tredition.de

Copyright:
The content of this book is sourced from the public domain.

The intention of the TREDITION CLASSICS series is to make world literature in the public domain available in printed format. Literary enthusiasts and organizations worldwide have scanned and digitally edited the original texts. tredition has subsequently formatted and redesigned the content into a modern reading layout. Therefore, we cannot guarantee the exact reproduction of the original format of a particular historic edition. Please also note that no modifications have been made to the spelling, therefore it may differ from the orthography used today.

Entered according to Act of Congress, in the year 1857, by
William Radde,
In the Clerk's Office of the District Court of the United States,
for the Southern District of New-York.

PREFACE.

In offering this pamphlet to the Public in general, and to Parents and Physicians in particular, I have no other object than that of contributing my share to the barrier which the medical profession has attempted, for more than two hundred years, to raise against the progress of the terrible disease which carries off upon an average, half a million of human beings annually. All the efforts of medical men to stop the ravages of Scarlet-Fever have hitherto proved unavailing; every remedy which was considered, for a while, a specific proved subsequently inefficient; and, notwithstanding the assertion to the contrary of a few, the Dr. Jenner who shall discover a reliable prophylactic against scarlatina, is probably not yet born. The patients die in the same proportion as they did two hundred and fifty years ago, and the physicians who have any success at all in the treatment of the terrible scourge, are those who treat for symptoms and leave the disease to Nature.

Under these circumstances, a mode of treatment which promises a decrease in the number of victims, from the experience of a quarter of a [Pg iv] century, and a score of epidemics of different characters, cannot but be received with pleasure by the public. I have treated scarlet-fever hydriatically for twenty-one years, and out of several hundred cases never lost a patient, except one who died of typhus during an epidemy of scarlatina; and my observations, during twenty-five years, of the practice of other physicians of the same school, present a result about as favorable as my own.

My present position is such, that no self-interest, if I could have any in a question of such importance for the human race; would induce me to publish this article, as a rush of scarlet-fever patients would only tend to destroy the practice at my establishment, instead of increasing my income. My purpose, therefore, must be honest; and the zeal which I have manifested for many years in the promulgation of the Water-Cure is no longer the effect of enthusiasm, but of the observations and practice of Priessnitz's method during the best part of a man's life, and the conviction of its merits gained from *facts*.

I consider Hydro-therapeutics as one of the healthiest branches of the Tree of Medical Science, but not, like some others do, as the whole Tree. I do not pretend to be able to cure every thing with water; but in yielding to other medical systems what belongs to them, I earnestly claim for the Water-Cure, what belongs to it, frankly accusing for the little progress the hydriatic system has made in this country, the spirit of charlatanism and speculation on one side, and ignorance, self-conceit, self-interest and laziness on the other. [Pg v] According to my experience, and the result obtained by other hydriatic practitioners, eruptive fevers decidedly belong to Hydro-therapeutics, or the Water-Cure. If the result obtained by men like Currie, Bateman, Gregory, Reuss, Frœlichsthal, &c., long before Priessnitz, were highly satisfactory, the important additions and the more systematic arrangement of the treatment of the inventor of the Water-Cure and myself, have made the method almost infallible in eruptive fevers, and my innermost conviction is, that all the other modes of treatment of these fevers put together will not do the tenth part of the service which may with certainty be expected from the systematic use of water as I give it in this treatise.

Owing to the reluctance of the profession to allow Hydro-therapeutics an honorable place among medical systems, I address myself more to parents than to physicians. Had I intended to write for the latter, exclusively, the important subject which I am treating, would have received another coat. However, nothing of value to the physician has been omitted, whilst much has been said, which though *he* does not need it, seemed to me indispensably necessary for people not initiated in the medical art.

In regard to the style and language in general, I solicit the reader's indulgence. I may appear pretentious in publishing the present pamphlet, written in a tongue which is not my own, without submitting it, previously, to the correction of an English or American pen; but this publication has been called forth by the tears of mothers mourning over the bodies of their [Pg vi] darlings during the present winter, and too much time has been lost already in preparing it, for those whose life might have been saved, by an earlier publication, whilst I am fully aware of the imperfections of a work, which has been done during the few, often interrupted, leisure-hours left to me by the position I occupy. But whatever may be its defects, I feel convinced, that it cannot fail doing some little good; and should but one mother's tears remain unshed, I would never regret having published it. The good it will do, must depend on the favor with which it is received.

CHARLES MUNDE.

Florence Water-Cure,}
  Northampton, Mass. }
March, 1857.

TABLE OF CONTENTS.

PART THE FIRST.
DESCRIPTION OF SCARLET-FEVER.

1. Definition—Scarlet-Fever or Scarlatina
2. Division of the process of the disease into *Periods*
3. Period of Incubation, or Hatching
4. Period of Eruption, or Appearing of the Rash
5. Period of Efflorescence, or Standing out of the Rash
6. Period of Desquamation, or Peeling off
7. Period of Convalescence
8. Varieties of Forms of Scarlatina
9. *Scarlatina simplex*, or simple Scarlet-Fever
10. *Scarlatina anginosa*, or Sore-Throat Scarlet-Fever
11. Mild Reaction (erethic)
12. Violent Reaction (sthenic)
13. Torpid Reaction (asthenic)
14. Scarlatina miliaris
15. Scarlatina sine Exanthemate
16. *Malignant Forms of Scarlatina*
17. Sudden Invasion of the Nervous Centres
18. Affection of the Brain
19.-20. Affection of the Cerebellum and Spine
21. Putrid Symptoms
22. Condition of the Throat, and other Internal Organs
23. Other bad symptoms
24. Destruction of the Organ of Hearing

25.	Other Sequels, Dropsy, &c.	
26.-27.	The *Contagion* of Scarlatina very active	
28.	*Diagnosis*	
29.	Diagnosis from Measles	
30.	*Prognosis*	
31.	Favorable symptoms	
32.	Unfavorable symptoms	

PART THE SECOND.
TREATMENT OF SCARLET-FEVER.

33.	*Different Methods of other Schools*	27
34.	The Expletive Method	
35.	The Anti-gastric Method	
36.	Ammonium carbonicum	
37.	Chloride of Lime	
38.	Acetic Acid	
39.	Mineral Acids. Muriatic Acids — Prescriptions	
40.	Frictions with Lard	
41.	Belladonna	
42.	There is neither a Specific nor a Prophylactic to be relied on	
43.	*Water-Treatment*, as used by Currie, Reuss, Hesse, Schœnlein, &c.	
44.	Priessnitz's Method — The wet-sheet-Pack	
45.-47.	Technicalities of the Pack and Bath	
48.	Action of the Pack and Bath — Rationale	
49.-50.	What effect could be expected from a warm wet-sheet?	
51.	No cutting short of the process of Scarlatina — the mor-	

11

bid poison must be drawn to the skin as soon as possible

52. Necessity of Ventilation — Means of Heating the sick-room — Relative merits of Open Fires, Stoves and Furnaces
53. Temperature of the sick-room
54. Water-drinking
55. Diet
56. *Treatment of Scarlatina simplex*
57. *Treatment of Scarlatina anginosa*
58.-65. *Treatment* of the *mild*, or erethic *Form* of scarlatina anginosa
66. *Treatment* of the *violent*, or sthenic *Form* of scarlatina anginosa
67. Temperature of the water — double sheet — Changing sheet
68.-69. Length of Pack — Perspiration
70. Length of Bath
71. Caution
72. The wet Compress
73. Highly inflamed Throat — Croup
74. Necessity of allaying the Heat
75.-77. The Half-bath — The Sitz- or Hip-Bath
78. Action of the sitz-bath explained
79.-80. Relaxation of Treatment towards the end of the third period — Continuation of Packs during and after Desquamation
81. Treatment of *torpid Forms* of scarlatina — Difference in the Treatment pointed out
82. Length of Pack
83. Cold Affusions and Rubbing

84. Ice-Water and Snow-Bath in malignant cases
85. Wine and Water, &c., if no reaction can be obtained
86. Ablutions and Rubbing with Iced-Water or Snow
87. Wet Compress
88. Ventilation all-important
89. Continuation of Packs—Convalescence
90. Mineral Acids, in case of severe sore Throat
91. Putrid Symptoms—Gargle—Solution of Chloride of Soda —Drink: Chlorate of potass—Liquor calcii chloridi
92. *Treatment of Affections of the Nervous Centres*
93.-94. Sitz-bath, anchor of safety
95.-97. Cases
98.-99. Impossibility of answering for the issue of every typhoid case
100. Is Water applicable in all typhoid cases?
101.-109. Rules for the application of water in typhoid cases
110.-112. Illustrations

PART THE THIRD.

113. *Treatment of other Eruptive Fevers*
114. Smalll-Pox
115. Varioloids, and Chicken-pocks
116. Measles
117. Urticaria, Zoster, Rubeola
118. Erysipelas
119. Erythema

120.- Additional Rules for the Treatment of Eruptive Diseas-
121. es
122. *Conclusive Remarks* — Obstacles
123. Want of Water
124. Dripping Sheet, substitute for the Half-bath
125. Rubbing Sheet, substitute for the Half-bath
126. Where there is a will, there is a way
127. Prejudice of Physicians against the Water-Cure
128. Rebellion!
129.- Facts
130.
131. More Facts!
132. Conclusion: Help yourselves, if your physicians will not help you!

PART I.

DESCRIPTION OF SCARLET-FEVER.

1. SCARLET-FEVER, OR SCARLATINA, [1]

is an eruptive fever, produced by a peculiar contagious poison, and distinguished by extreme heat, a rapid pulse, a severe affection of the mucous membranes, especially those of the mouth and throat, and by a burning scarlet eruption on the skin.

2. DIVISION OF THE PROCESS OF THE DISEASE INTO PERIODS.

Its course is commonly divided into four distinct periods, viz.: the period of incubation, the period of eruption, the period of efflorescence, and the period of desquamation; to which may be added: the period of convalescence.

3. PERIOD OF INCUBATION, OR HATCHING.

The time which passes between the reception of the contagious poison into the system and the appearance of the rash, is called the period of incubation; incubation or incubus meaning, properly, the sitting of birds on their nests, and figuratively, the hatching or concoction of the poison within the body, until prepared for its elimination. There is no certainty about the time necessary for that purpose, as the contagion, after the patient has come [Pg 14] in contact with it, may be lurking a longer or a shorter time about his person, or in his clothes and furniture.

As in almost all eruptive fevers, so in scarlatina, the patient begins with complaining of shivering, pain in the thighs, lassitude, and rapidly augmenting debility; frequently also of headache, which, when severe, is accompanied with delirium, nausea and vomiting. The fever soon becomes very high, the pulse increasing to upwards of 120 to 130 strokes in a minute, and more; the heat is extreme, raising the natural temperature of the body from 98 to 110-112 degrees Fahrenheit, being intenser internally than on the surface of the body. The patient complains of severe pain in the throat, the organs of deglutition located there becoming inflamed, and swelling to such a degree that swallowing is extremely difficult, and even breathing is impeded. The tongue is covered with a white creamy coat, through which the points of the elongated papillæ project. Gradually the white coat disappears, commencing at the end and the edges of the organ, and leaves the same in a clean, raw, inflamed state, looking much like a huge strawberry. This is called the *strawberry tongue* of scarlet-fever, and is one of the characteristic symptoms of that disease. There is a peculiar smell about the person of the patient, reminding one of salt fish, old cheese, or the cages of a menagerie.

4. PERIOD OF ERUPTION, OR APPEARING OF THE RASH.

Commonly, on the second day, towards evening, sometimes on the third, and only in very bad cases later, the rash begins to make its appearance, under an increase of the above symptoms, especially of the fever and delirium, and continues to come out for about twelve hours. Usually the eruption commences in the face, on the throat and chest; thence it spreads over the rest of the trunk, and finally it extends to the extremities. The minute [Pg 15] red points, which appear at first, soon spread into large, flat, irregular patches, which again coalesce and cover the greater part, if not the whole, of the surface, being densest on the upper part of the body, particularly in front, in the face, on the neck, the inner side of the arms, the loins, and the bend of the joints. The scarlet color of the rash disappears under the pressure of the finger, but reappears immediately on the latter being removed. Sometimes the eruption takes place with a profuse warm sweat, which prognosticates a mild course and a favorable issue of the disorder. Together with the appearance of the rash, the disease develops itself also more internally: the inflammation of the mouth and throat increases; the tonsils and fauces swell to a high degree; the eyes become suffused and sensitive to the light; the mucous membranes of the nose and bronchia become also affected, the patient sneezes and coughs, and all the symptoms denote the intense struggle, in which the whole organism is engaged, to rid itself of the enemy which has taken possession of it.

5. PERIOD OF EFFLORESCENCE, OR STANDING OUT OF THE RASH.

During the first day or two of the period of efflorescence, which lasts three or four days, the above symptoms usually continue to increase. Sometimes, however, the patient is alleviated at once on the rash being formed. This alleviation always takes place when the rash comes with perspiration, and also under a proper course of water-treatment. If the rash continues to stand out steadily, the symptoms decrease on the third day; the patient becomes more quiet, the pulse slower (going down to 90 and even to 80 strokes per minute); the rash, then, gradually and steadily fades, and finally disappears altogether.—Sometimes the rash fades or disappears too early, in which cases, usually, the internal symptoms [Pg 16] increase, the brain and spine become affected, and the situation of the patient becomes critical.

6. PERIOD OF DESQUAMATION, OR PEELING-OFF.

About the sixth or seventh day, the epidermis, or cuticle of the skin begins to peal off, commencing in those places which first became the seat of the rash, and gradually continuing all over the body. In such parts as are covered with a thin delicate cuticle (as the face, breast, &c.) the cuticle comes off in small dry scurfs; in such parts as are covered with a thicker epidermis, in large flakes. There have been instances of almost complete gloves and slippers coming away from patients' hands and feet.—The fever subsides entirely, and so does the inflammation of the throat and mouth, which become moist again. Also the epithelia, or the delicate cuticles of the mucous membranes, which have been affected by the disease, peal off and are coughed up with the tough thick mucus covering the throat, or they are evacuated with the fæces and the urine, forming a sediment in the latter.—Desquamation is usually completed in from three to five days; sometimes it requires a longer time; under hydriatic treatment it seldom lasts more than a few days. Whilst desquamation is taking place, a new cuticle forms itself, which, being exceedingly thin at first, gives the patient a redder color than usual for some time, and requires him to be cautious, in order to prevent bad consequences from exposure.—

Thus the disease makes its regular course in about ten days, and, under a course of hydriatic treatment, which not only assists the organism in throwing off the morbid poison and keeps the patient in good condition, but also protects him from the influence of the atmosphere, the patient may consider himself out of danger and leave the sick-room under proper caution, of which we shall speak hereafter.

[Pg 17]

7. THE PERIOD OF CONVALESCENCE,

under the usual drug-treatment, is, however, usually protracted to twice or thrice the duration of the disease, the patient being compelled to keep the house for five or six weeks, especially from fear of *anasarca*, or dropsy of the skin, frequently extending to the inner cavities of the body, and proving fatal. This dangerous complaint has been more frequently observed after mild cases of scarlet-fever than after malignant cases, probably from the fact that in mild cases the patient is more apt to expose himself, than when the danger is more obvious and all possible care is taken.—Sometimes also severe rheumatic pain, or rather neuralgia, in the joints, swelling of the glands, and other sequels prolong his sickness. I never observed a case of dropsy, or of neuralgia, after a course of water-treatment.

8. VARIETIES OF FORMS OF SCARLATINA.

The above is the description of scarlet-fever, as it most frequently occurs. But far from taking always that regular course, the constitution of the patient, the intensity of the epidemy and the virulence of the poison, the treatment and other circumstances influencing the development of the disease, cause several anomalies, from scarlatina simplex to scarlatina maligna, which too often baffles all the resources of the Medical Art.

9. SCARLATINA SIMPLEX, OR SIMPLE SCARLET-FEVER.

In the *mildest form* of the disease, called *scarlatina simplex*, or *simple scarlet-fever*, there is no inflammation of the throat, the fever is moderate, and the patient suffers very little. Unfortunately this form is so rare, that many experienced physicians never saw a case. Probably, it was a case belonging to this class, which was mentioned a number of years ago by one of the writers on Priessnitz's practice, when a lady with [Pg 18] scarlet-fever joined a dancing party at Græfenberg, a case for reporting which the author [2] has been ridiculed by the opponents of the Water-Cure, but which by no means belongs to impossibilities; for scarlatina simplex having been declared by eminent physicians (not of Priessnitz's school) to be "scarcely a disease," [3] becoming fatal only through the officiousness of the doctor, [4] and other physicians of note recommending cold rooms and open air through the whole course of the disease, [5] or at least towards the latter part of it; [6] I do not see why a patient under water-treatment should not be safer in producing perspiration by dancing than in sitting in a cold room or in walking in the open street. The fact, of course, is unusual, and I do not exactly recommend its practice, but it is not at all impossible, and ridiculing the reporter of it shows either ignorance of the disease or a bad will towards the new curative system, to which those are most opposed who know the least of it.

10. SCARLATINA ANGINOSA, OR SORE-THROAT SCARLET-FEVER.

Wherever the *throat* is affected, which is almost always the case, the disease is called *scarlatina anginosa*, or *sore-throat scarlet-fever*.

This is the form described at the commencement of this article. There are several varieties, however, of scarlatina anginosa.

In any case, the organism, invaded by the contagious poison, will try to rid itself of its enemy. The reaction is necessarily in proportion to the violence of the miasma and to the quantity of organic power struggling against it.

[Pg 19]

11. MILD REACTION (ERETHIC).

If the poison is not virulent, and the body of the patient in a favorable condition, the *reaction* is *mild*, and the poison is eliminated without any violent efforts on the part of the organism. This is the case in scarlatina simplex, and in mild forms of scarlatina anginosa.

12. VIOLENT REACTION (STHENIC).

If both, the contagious poison and the organism, are very strong, a *violent reaction* will take place, and the safety of the patient will be endangered by the very violence of the struggle, by which internal organs may be more or less affected.

13. TORPID REACTION (ASTHENIC).

The more violent the contagious poison, and the weaker the organic power, the less decidedly and the less successfully will the organism combat against the poison, and the more inroad will the latter make upon the system, affecting vital organs and paralyzing the efforts of the nervous system by attacking it in its centres. In such cases of *torpid reaction*, the patient frequently passes at once into a *typhoid state*. This is what we call *scarlatina maligna*, or *malignant scarlet-fever*.

14. SCARLATINA MILIARIS

Sometimes the red patches of the rash are covered with small vesicles of the size of mustard-seed, which either dry up or discharge a watery liquid, leaving thin white scurfs, that come away with the cuticle during desquamation. Although this form, called *scarlatina miliaris*, being the result of exudation from the capillary vessels, shows an intensely inflamed state of the skin, its course is usually mild and its issue favorable; because the morbid poison comes readily to the surface.

[Pg 20]

15. SCARLATINA SINE EXANTHEMATE.

There are also mild cases of scarlet-fever, when little or no rash appears, and the throat is very little affected. These are the result of a particularly mild character of the epidemy, together with a peculiar condition of the skin, the desquamation of which shows that the poison went to the surface without producing the usual state of inflammation, or the rash peculiar to the disease. This form, called *scarlatina sine exanthemate*, is extremely rare.

16. THE MALIGNANT FORMS OF SCARLET-FEVER

are caused by the character of the epidemy, but, perhaps, more frequently by the weak and sickly constitution of the patient and the external circumstances affecting it. Thus, persons of scrofulous habit, being naturally of a low organization, without much power of resistance, are much more liable to experience the destructive effects of scarlatina than those whose organism possesses sufficient energy to resist the action of the morbid poison, and to expel it before it can do any serious harm inside the body.

17. SUDDEN INVASION OF THE NERVOUS CENTRES.

Of the different forms of scarlatina maligna the most dangerous is the sudden invasion of the nervous system, particularly the *brain*, the *cerebellum* and the *spine*, by which the patient's life is sometimes extinguished in a few hours. In other cases the symptoms deepen more gradually, and death ensues on the third, fifth or seventh day.

18. AFFECTION OF THE BRAIN.

When the *brain* is affected, the patient suddenly complains of violent headache, vomits repeatedly, loses his eye-sight, has furious delirium, or coma (a state of sleep from which it is difficult to rouse the patient); his [Pg 21] pupils dilate; the pulse becomes small, intermits; sometimes the skin becomes cold; there is dyspnœa (difficulty of breathing), fainting, paralysis, convulsions, and finally death; or, sometimes, the paroxysm passes suddenly by with bleeding from the nose or with a profuse perspiration.

19. AFFECTION OF THE CEREBELLUM AND SPINE.

In affections of the *cerebellum* and *spinal marrow*, the patient complains of violent pain in the back of the head and neck, in the spine, and frequently in the whole body. These also frequently terminate with the destruction of life.

20. During all these invasions of the nervous centres there is little or no rash, and what appears is of a pale, livid hue.

21. PUTRID SYMPTOMS.

Next to those most dangerous forms—most dangerous, because the organic power (the *vis medicatrix naturæ*), from which the restoration of health must be expected, and without which no physician can remove the slightest symptom of disease, becomes partly paralyzed from the beginning—*putrid symptoms* present a good deal of danger, although they give the organism and the physician more time to act.

22. CONDITION OF THE THROAT, AND OTHER INTERNAL ORGANS.

The condition of the *throat* requires the most constant attention. From a highly inflamed state, it often passes into a foul and sloughy condition; the breath of the patient becomes extremely fetid; the nostrils, the parotid and submaxillary glands swell enormously, so that swallowing and breathing become very difficult. There is an acrid discharge from the nose; the [Pg 22] gangrenous matter affects the alimentary canal, causing pain in the stomach, the bowels, the kidneys and the bladder; a smarting diarrhœa with excoriation of the anus, and inflammatory symptoms of the vulva. Also the bronchia, lungs, pleura and pericardium become affected, as sneezing, cough (the so-called scarlet-cough) and the pain across the chest and in the region of the heart indicate.

23. OTHER BAD SYMPTOMS.

These symptoms may present themselves with the rash standing out; but most frequently they occur when there is little or no eruption, or when it fades, becomes livid, or disappears altogether. A sudden disappearance of the rash, before the sixth day, commonly increases the typhoid symptoms, and must be considered a bad omen. Also the invasion of the larynx, which is happily of rare occurrence, is commonly fatal.

24. DESTRUCTION OF THE ORGAN OF HEARING.

When the glands pass into a sloughing state, the parts connected with them are frequently damaged. Thus the ulceration of the parotid gland often causes deafness, by the gangrenous matter communicating to the eustachian tube and the inner ear, where it destroys the membrane of the drum and the little bones belonging thereto, or by closing up the tube. When the discharge from the outer ear is observed, the destruction has already taken place, and it is too late to obviate the injury.

25. OTHER SEQUELS, DROPSY, &C.

Beside the ulceration of glands and deafness, some of the sequels of scarlatina are white swelling of one or more of the joints, usually the knee, chronic inflammation of the eyes and eyelids, and partial paralysis. These chiefly occur in scrofulous subjects. Dropsy, which [Pg 23] I have mentioned before, is one of the sequels that frequently prove fatal.

26. THE CONTAGION OF SCARLATINA VERY ACTIVE.

The *contagion* of scarlatina is very active, and adheres for a long time to the sick-room, bedding, clothes and furniture. The best means to destroy it, is plenty of air. It is difficult to say when the contagion is over, as much depends on the season of the year and the care with which the house is aired. Physicians and visitors at the sick-room are very apt to carry it about, unless they be exceedingly careful in changing their clothes and washing themselves, hair and all, before entering other rooms inhabited by persons who had not had the disorder before. It is astonishing how easily such persons are taken by it; and it even sometimes happens that such as have gone through it, take it again in after years. I am authorized by experience, that the idea as if patients under water-treatment, or even such as take a cold bath every morning, were inaccessible to the contagion, is erroneous. I have had patients under treatment for chronic diseases, who had had scarlatina several years before, and neither this nor the water-cure protected them from taking it again. With some of them, however, the throat only became affected and no desquamation took place, whilst the character of the complaint with the rest was rather mild. I have been astonished to read that in a meeting of a medical society of this country, which took place a very short time ago, some members could have raised the question whether scarlatina was really contagious. I admit that the profession in general has not made great progress in the cure of the complaint, but it does not require great study and long experience to know that scarlet-fever is contagious!

27. The form of the disorder in one patient does not [Pg 24] imply the necessity of another who caught it from him having it in the same form. A person can take the contagion from one who dies of malignant scarlet-fever and have it in the mildest form, and vice versa. The character of the disease depends very much on the constitution, as I have said above. However, if the epidemy in general is of a malignant character (which may again depend, partly at least, on the constitution of the atmosphere), it will prove so in many individuals who are taken with it, and the precautions ought to be so much the more careful on that account.

28. DIAGNOSIS.

After what has been said about the symptoms of scarlatina, it cannot be difficult to distinguish it from similar eruptive diseases. However, as there is much resemblance between *scarlatina* and *measles*, at least in the milder form of the former, I shall give a few symptoms of each, to assist parents in making the distinction.

29. DIAGNOSIS FROM MEASLES.

In scarlatina the heat is much greater, and the pulse is much quicker than in measles. — In scarlatina the throat is inflamed, usually the brain affected, and the patient smells like salt-fish, old cheese or the cages of a menagerie; in measles, the eyes are affected, inflamed, and incapable of bearing the light; the organs of respiration likewise (thence coryza, sneezing, hoarseness, cough); the perspiration smells like the feathers of geese freshly plucked. — In scarlatina the period of incubation is a day less than in measles; namely, in scarlatina the rash appears on the second day after the first symptoms, in measles on the third. — The scarlet-rash consists of large, irregular, *flat* patches, which cover large spaces with a uniform scarlet-red, being brightest in those parts which are usually covered by the garments of the patient; [Pg 25] in measles the spots are small, roundish or half-moon-like, with little grains upon them, and usually of a darker color; the measle-rash is thickest in such parts as are exposed to the air.—In scarlatina the symptoms of fever and the affection of the mucous membranes continue two days after the eruption has begun to make its appearance; in measles the eruption diminishes those symptoms at once.—The scarlet-rash stands out a day or two less than the measle-rash, and comes off in laminæ, whilst the latter comes off in small scales or scurfs.

30. THE PROGNOSIS,

under a well conducted course of hydriatic treatment is, in general, favorable. Much depends, however, on the season of the year (in damp and cold weather—partly owing to a lack of pure air in the sick-room—the disease is more dangerous than in summer); on the general health of the patient (not on his mere looks, for well-fed and stout children are subject to affections of the brain); on the age of the patient (adults are generally more in danger than children); on the form of the disease and the character of the fever (erethic or mild fever being the most favorable, whilst typhoid fever is the worst; a violent character of the fever is not very dangerous under hydriatic treatment, as we have plenty of means to limit its ravages without weakening the patient); on the eruption, the condition of the throat, the process of desquamation, &c.

31. FAVORABLE SYMPTOMS

are the following: Absence of internal inflammation; a bright florid rash; a regular, steady appearance, standing out, and disappearance of the latter; a regular and complete pealing off of the cuticle; a decrease of the pulse after the eruption of the rash; an easy and regular [Pg 26] respiration; a natural expression of the features; a moist skin.

32. UNFAVORABLE SYMPTOMS

are: A fetid breath, with ulceration and sloughing of the throat and glands; a smarting and weakening diarrhœa; involuntary evacuations of the bowels; dizziness, deafness, coma, grinding of the teeth; retention of urine; petechiæ; a rapid decline of the patient's strength; a quick, small, weak pulse; rapid breathing; twitchings, tetanus, hiccough, &c.—Closing up of the nose frequently precedes a dangerous affection of the brain. A sudden disappearance of the rash, or of the inflammation of the throat, is a bad omen. With such symptoms as these, there is usually little or no rash, and the little there is, of a pale, livid color, and the skin, in general, inactive.

FOOTNOTES:

[1] The expression *scarlatina* does not imply, as it is believed by many, on account of its diminutive form, a peculiar mild form of the disease: it is nothing but the Latin and scientific name for scarlet-fever.

[2] Captain Claridge.

[3] Thomas Watson, M. D. Lectures on the Principles and Practice of Physic.

[4] Sydenham.

[5] G. C. Reich, M.D. Neue Aufschluesse ueber die Natur und Heilung des Scharlachfiebers, Halle, 1810.

[6] L. Hesse, M. D. in Rust's Magazin, Vol. XXVII., H. 1 S. 109.

[Pg 27]

PART II.

TREATMENT OF SCARLET-FEVER.

DIFFERENT METHODS OF OTHER SCHOOLS.

33. Before giving the description of hydriatic treatment of scarlet-fever, I shall, for the sake of a better appreciation, glance over the different methods which have been recommended by other schools.

34. THE EXPLETIVE METHOD (*blood-letting*)

has been advocated by some of the best authorities, and there cannot be a doubt but that it must have rendered good service in cases of violent reaction, or else men like de Haen, Wendt, Willan, Morton, Alcock, Dewees, Dawson, Dewar, Hammond, &c., would not have pronounced themselves in favor of it. However it requires nice discrimination and a great deal of experience, as in any case where it does no good it is apt to do a great deal of harm, by weakening the patient and thus depriving him of that power which he so much needs in struggling against the enemy invading his system. Besides, the expletive method has found many antagonists of weight: Simon, Williams, Tweedie, Allison and others have shown the danger of a general and indiscriminate use of it. Williams, [7] in his comparison of the epidemics of scarlatina from 1763 to 1834, has come to the conclusion that the possibility of a cure in cases of blood-letting, compared with the cases where the patients have not been bled, is like [Pg 28] 1:4; i. e. four patients have died after blood-letting, when only one died without bleeding. "Experience has equally shown, says Dr. Allison, that the expectation entertained by Dr. Armstrong [8] and others, that by early depletion the congestive or malignant form of the disease may be made to assume the more healthy form of inflammation and fever, is hardly ever realized; and in many cases, although the pulse has been full and the eruption florid in the beginning, *blood-letting (even local blood-letting) has been followed by a rapid change of the fever to a typhoid type, and manifestly aggravated the danger."* —My own experience would prompt me to declare myself against blood-letting in general, even if I had not a sufficient quantity of water at hand to manage the violent or irregular reaction of a case. Blood-letting, in any case of eruptive fever, and with few exceptions in almost every other case, appears to me like pulling down the house to extinguish the fire. A little experience in hydriatics, a few buckets of water, with a couple of linen sheets and blankets, will answer all the indications and remove the danger without sending the patient from Scylla into Charybdis.

35. THE ANTI-GASTRIC METHOD,

consisting in the free use of emetics or purgatives, has been recommended by some eminent practitioners. Withering, [9] Tissot, Kennedy and others are in favor of the former, and find fault with the latter, whilst Hamilton, [10] Willard, Abernethy, Gregory, &c., prefer purgatives, and some, of course, look upon calomel as the anchor of safety, which they recommend in quantities of from five to ten grains per hour. [11] The friends of one part of the [Pg 29] anti-gastric method make war upon the other: Withering finding purgatives entirely out of place and Sandwith, Fothergill and others having seen nothing but harm done by them, whilst Wendt, [12] Berndt, [13] Heyfelder and others caution their readers against emetics. The anti-gastric method has been of some service in epidemics and individual cases, when the character of the disease was decidedly gastric and bilious. To use emetics or purgatives indiscriminately would do much more harm than good; as, for instance, during a congestive condition of the brain, the former, and with inflammatory symptoms of the bowels, the latter, would be almost sure to sacrifice the patient to the method.

36. THE AMMONIUM CARBONICUM,

recommended by Peart, [14] has been considered by many as a specific capable of neutralizing the scarlatinous poison, whilst others have used it only as a powerful tonic in torpid cases. Experience has shown that it is not a specific, and that its use as a tonic, requiring a great deal of care and discrimination, is a good deal more dangerous than the mode of treatment I am going to recommend in cases where tonics are required.

37. CHLORIDE OF LIME.

About the same opinion may be given on *Chloride of Lime*. As a gargle, and taken internally, the aqua-chlorina has done good service in malignant scarlatina, especially in putrid cases.

38. ACETIC ACID.

Brown [15] recommends diluted *Acetic Acid* as a specific against all forms of scarlatina. Experience, however, has not supported his confidence in the infallibility of his remedy.

39. MINERAL ACIDS (MURIATIC ACID – PRESCRIPTIONS)

have also been used with good effect in some epidemics. *Muriatic acid* I have frequently used myself for inflammation of the throat, in connection with hydriatic treatment, and it has almost always contributed to relieve the symptoms materially. [16]

40. FRICTIONS WITH LARD

were used already by Cælius Aurelianus, [17] and recently reintroduced into practice, by Drs. Dæne and Schneemann, [18] in Germany, and by Dr. Lindsley, [19] in America. Even hydriatic physicians [20] have tried them with some success. However, notwithstanding the strong recommendations of the remedy on the part of the above named practitioners and others, the efficacy of it as a general remedy for scarlet-fever has not been confirmed. On the contrary, Berend [21] and Hauner [22] found that it did not prevent desquamation, as it had been asserted, and even Richter restricts his commendations to the vague assertion "that it seemed to him as if the cases when he used the lard were made milder than they would have been without it."

41. BELLADONNA.

The remedy which has attracted and still attracts in a very high degree the attention of physicians and parents, is *Belladonna*. This remedy was first introduced as a specific and prophylactic by Hahnemann, and soon recommended not only by his own disciples, but by some of the best names of the "regular" school. [23] But soon after, as many physicians of standing declared themselves adversaries to Hahnemann's discovery, [24] and whatever may be the merits of belladonna as a specific and prophylactic in some quarters, it is certain that it never answered the expectation raised by its promulgators in others. As far as my own experience extends, I have seen very little or no effect from it. I have restricted myself, it is true, to homœopathic doses, being afraid of the bad consequences of larger quantities in children; but from what I have seen in my own practice and that of some other physicians with whom I was familiar, I cannot but advise my readers not *to rely* either on the [Pg 32] prophylactic or the curative power of belladonna, when a safer and more reliable remedy is offered to them. A remedy may be excellent in certain cases and certain epidemics, and many an honest and well-meaning physician may be deceived into the belief that he has a general remedy in hand, whilst others, or himself, on future occasions discover that he has allowed himself to be taken in. Had not belladonna and aconite proved beneficial in many cases, they would scarcely have acquired their reputation, but with all due respect for Father Hahnemann and his system, I must deny belladonna to be a general, safe and reliable remedy in the prevention and cure of scarlet-fever.

42. THERE IS NEITHER A SPECIFIC NOR A PROPHYLACTIC TO BE RELIED ON.

All these different methods and remedies, and many others, have been and are still used with more or less effect. But where there are three physicians to recommend one of them, there will always be four to contradict them. They may all do some good in certain epidemics or individual cases; they may relieve symptoms; they may save the life of many a patient who would have died without them (although many a patient who died, might have lived also, had he been under a more judicious treatment, or—under no treatment at all.) But none is reliable in general; none contains a specific to neutralize the morbid poison; none is a reliable prophylactic, such as vaccina for small-pox; and if single physicians, or whole classes of physicians, assert to the contrary, the fault must lie somewhere, either in their excess of faith in certain authorities, which induces them to throw their own pia desideria into the scales, or in a want of cool, impartial observation continued for a sufficient length of time to wear out sanguine expectations. *The fact is that there neither exists a reliable [Pg 33] prophylactic, nor has a safe specific been found as yet; that all is guess-and-piece work; and that people are taken by scarlet-fever and die of it about the same as before those vaunted methods and remedies were discovered.* I wish to impress my readers with this fact—the proofs of which they can easily find in the mortality lists of the papers—to make them understand that by giving up for the hydriatic method any of the modes and remedies, which have been in use hitherto, they do not run a risk of losing anything.

43. WATER-TREATMENT, AS USED BY CURRIE, REUSS, HESSE, SCHŒNLEIN, &C.

Beside the above modes of treatment *cold* and *tepid Water* has been extensively used and recommended by reliable authorities. Currie, [25] Pierce, Gregory, Bateman, von Wedekind, Kolbany, [26] Torrence, Reuss, [27] von Fröhlichsthal, [28] and others, have treated their scarlet-patients with *cold affusions*. Henke, Raimann, Fröhlich, Hesse, [29] Steimmig, [30] Gregory, Jr., Schœnlein, Fuchs, and others, have not ventured beyond *cool* and *tepid ablutions*. The former, although the general result has been very satisfactory, have proved dangerous in some cases; and the latter, though safer in general, have not been efficient in many others. The use of water, though safer than other remedies, has never become general, *owing to the unsystematic, unsafe, or inefficient forms of its application.*

[Pg 34] Fear and prejudice—fed by the great mass of physicians, who generally take too much care of their reputation to expose it in the use of a remedy the effects of which are so easily understood by every one—have also been obstacles to its promulgation; and the exaggerations of some of its advocates in modern times, bearing for a great part the characteristics of charlatanism, have scared many who might have become converts to Priessnitz's method, to whose genius and good luck we are indebted for the most important, most harmless, and at the same time the most efficient and most reliable discovery, viz.:

44. PRIESSNITZ'S METHOD—THE WET-SHEET-PACK,

a remedy which, alone, is worth the whole antiphlogistic, diaphoretic, and, indeed, the whole curative apparatus of the profession, in ancient and modern times, for any kind of fevers, and especially for eruptive diseases. Nor did the physicians before Priessnitz know anything about the use of the *sitz-bath* for affections of the brain in torpid reaction, which in such cases, is the only anchor of safety. In short, water-treatment was, like other methods, an excellent thing for certain symptoms, but not generally and safely applicable in every case.

To appreciate the effects of the wet-sheet pack, one must have seen it used for inflammatory fever, when it acts like a charm, frequently removing all the feverish symptoms, and their cause, in a few hours.

45. TECHNICALITIES OF THE PACK AND BATH.

Let me give you its technicalities, and the rationale of its action:

A linen sheet, (linen is a better conductor than cotton,) large enough to wrap the whole person of the patient in it (not too large, however; if there is no sheet of proper size, it should be doubled at the upper end) is dipped in water of a temperature answering to the degree of heat [Pg 35] and fever, say between fifty and seventy degrees Fahrenheit, and more or less tightly wrung out. The higher the temperature of the body, and the quicker and fuller the pulse, the lower the temperature of the water, and the wetter the sheet. This wet sheet is spread upon a blanket previously placed on the mattress of the bed on which the packing is to take place. The patient, wholly undressed, is laid upon it, stretched out in all his length, and his arms close to his thighs, and quickly wrapped up in the sheet, head and all, with the exception of the face; the blanket is thrown over the sheet, first on the packer's side, folded down about the head and shoulders, so as to make it stick tight to all parts of the body, especially the neck and feet, tucked under the shoulders, side of the trunk, leg and foot; then the opposite side of the blanket is folded and tucked under in the same manner, till the blanket and sheet cover the whole body *smoothly* and *tightly*. Then comes a feather-bed, or a comforter doubled up, and packed on and around the patient, so that no heat can escape, or air enter in any part of the pack, if the head be very hot, it may be left out of the pack, or the sheet may be doubled around it, or a cold wet compress, not too much wrung out, be placed on the forehead, and as far back on the top of the head as practicable, which compress must be changed from time to time, to keep it cool. Thus the patient remains.

46. The first impression of the cold wet sheet is disagreeable; but no sooner does the blanket cover the sheet, than the chill passes away, and usually before the packing is completed, the patient begins to feel more comfortable, and very soon the symptoms of the fever diminish. The pulse becomes softer, slower, the breathing easier, the head cooler, the general irritation is allayed, and frequently the patient shows some inclination to sleep. When the fever and heat are very high, the [Pg 36] sheet must be changed on growing hot, as then it would cause the symptoms to increase again, instead of continuing to relieve them. The best way to effect this changing of the sheet is to prepare another blanket and sheet on another bed, to unpack the patient and carry him to the new pack,

where the process described above is repeated. Sometimes it is necessary to change again; but seldom more than three sheets are required to produce a perspiration, and relieve the patient for several hours, or—according to the case—permanently. The changing of the sheet may become necessary in fifteen, twenty, twenty-five, thirty or forty minutes, according to the degree of fever and heat. In every new sheet the patient can stay longer; in the last sheet he becomes more quiet than before, usually falls asleep, and awakes in a profuse perspiration, which carries off the alarming symptoms.

47. A few minutes before the perspiration breaks out, the patient becomes slightly irritated, which irritation is removed by the appearance of the sweat. I mention this circumstance, to prevent his being taken out just before the perspiration is started. When he becomes restless *during perspiration*, he is taken from his pack and placed in a bathing-tub partly filled with cool or tepid water, (usually of about 70°,) which has been prepared in the meanwhile; there he is washed down from head to foot, water from the bath being constantly thrown over him until he becomes cool. Then he is wrapped in a dry sheet, gently rubbed dry, and either taken back to his bed, or dressed and allowed to walk about the room. When the fever and heat rise again, the same process is repeated.

48. ACTION OF THE PACK AND BATH.—RATIONALE.

The action of the wet-sheet pack is thus easily accounted for:

[Pg 37] According to a well-known physical law, any cold body, whether dead or alive, placed in close contact with a warm body, will abstract from the latter as much heat as necessary to equalize the temperature of both. The transfer of caloric will begin at the place at which the two bodies are nearest to each other. The wet sheet, which touches the patient's body all over the surface, abstracts heat from the latter, till the temperature of the sheet becomes equal to that of the body. In proportion as the surface of the body yields heat to the sheet, the parts next to the surface impart heat to the latter, and so forth, till the whole body becomes cooler, whilst the sheet becomes warmer. As the heat imparted to the sheet cannot escape from it, the sheet being closely wrapt up in the blanket and bed, the current of caloric once established towards every part of the surface of the body will still continue; after the temperature of the sheet and the body has become equal, there will be an accumulation of heat around the body, frequently of a higher degree than the body itself. To explain this phenomenon, we ought to consider that we have not to do with *two dead* bodies, but with *one dead* and *one living* body, which constantly creates heat, thus continuously supplying the heat escaping from it to the sheet, and keeping up the current of caloric *and electricity* established towards the surface. There cannot be a doubt that the abstraction of electricity from the feverish organism contributes in a great measure to the relief of the excited nerves of the patient, as well as to the excess of temperature observed around the body in the wet-sheet pack (after the patient has been in it for some time); and that, in general, electricity deserves a closer investigation in the morbid phenomena of the human body than it has found to this day.

[Pg 38] 49. WHAT EFFECT COULD BE EXPECTED FROM A WARM WET-SHEET?

The first impression of the wet-sheet is, as I stated before, a *disagreeable* one. If it were *agreeable* — as a warm sheet, for instance, would be, which has been occasionally tried, of course without doing any good — *it would not produce a reaction at all, and consequently there would be no relief for, and finally no cure of the patient effected by it.* But the impression of the cold sheet, being powerful, is transferred at once from the peripherical nerves, which receive the shock, to the nervous centres (the spine, the cerebellum and the brain), and, in fact, to the whole nervous system, and the reaction is almost immediate; the vascular system, participating in it, sends the blood from the larger vessels and the vital parts, to the capillaries of the skin; and when, through repeated applications of the sheet, the system is relieved and harmony restored, in a sufficient degree, in and among the different parts of the organism, to enable them to resume their partly impeded functions, a profuse perspiration brings the struggle to a close, by removing the morbid matter which caused the fever, whereupon the skin is refreshed and strengthened, and the whole body cooled and protected by a cool bath from obnoxious atmospheric influences.

50. I am not aware that a better rationale can be given of the action of other remedies. Any physician can understand that its effect must be at once powerful and safe, and that there is no risk in the wet-sheet pack of the reaction not taking place, as it may be the case in severer applications of cold water, without the pack. One objection I have often heard, viz.: that the process is very troublesome. But what does trouble signify, when the life and health of a fellow-being is at stake?—It is true, the physician is frequently compelled to [Pg 39] render the services of a bath-attendant, and stay with the patient much longer than in the usual practice; but he gets through sooner, and, if not the patient and his friends, his own conscience will pay him for his exertions and sacrifice of time.

There is little trouble with small children, who make a fuss only, and become refractory, when the parents, grandmammas and aunts set the example. When all remain quiet, and treat the whole proceeding as a matter of necessity, children usually submit to it very patiently, and soon become quiet, should they be excited at the beginning. The fewer words are said, and the quicker and firmer the physician performs the whole process, the less there is trouble. After having been taught how to do it, the parents or friends of the patient will be able to take the most troublesome part of the business off the physician's hands, who, of course, has more necessary things to do, during an epidemic, than to pack his patients and attend to them in all their baths himself.

Only with spoiled children I have had trouble, and more with them that spoiled them. The best course, then, is to retain only one person for assistance, and to send the rest away till all is over. There are people, who *will* be unreasonable; of course, it is no use to attempt reasoning with them. I remember the grandmother of a little patient, with whom the pack acted like a miracle, removing a severe inflammatory fever in two hours and a half, telling me "she would rather see the child die, than have her packed again," although she acknowledged the pack to have been the means of her speedy recovery. It is true there was some trouble with the child, but only because the whole family were assembled in the sick-room to excite the child through their unseasonable lamentations and expressions of sympathy about the "dreadful" treatment to which she was going to be submitted. Grandmother would not have objected [Pg 40] to a pound of calomel! — But we shall speak about objections and difficulties in a more proper place.

51. NO CUTTING SHORT OF THE PROCESS OF SCARLATINA — THE MORBID POISON MUST BE DRAWN TO THE SKIN AS SOON AS POSSIBLE.

Scarlet-fever is a disease, which cannot be cut short. Any attempt to stop the process of incubation, after the contagion has once been received within the body, or to prevent its being thrown out upon the surface, would destroy the patient's life: the morbid poison must be concocted, and it *must come away by being drawn to the skin as soon as possible*, to prevent its settling in the vital parts, and injuring them. The safest way of assisting nature in her efforts of eliminating the poison, is to open the way, which she points out herself. We know that the sooner and the more completely the eruption makes its appearance, the brighter and the more constant the rash, the less there is danger for the patient, and *vice versa*. Well, there is not a better remedy than the wet-sheet pack, to serve the purpose of nature, i. e., to remove the morbid poison from the inner organs, and draw it to the surface; whilst at the same time it allays the symptoms, improves the condition of the skin for the development of the rash, and relieves the patient, without depriving him of any part of that organic power so indispensable for a cure, and without which the best physician in the world becomes a mere blank. Under the process of wet-sheet packing, the heat invariably abates, the pulse becomes slower and softer, the violence of the symptoms is alleviated, the skin becomes moist, the restlessness and anxiety of the patient give way to a more quiet and comfortable condition; he perspires and falls in a refreshing sleep. Is there any other remedy, that has the same general and beneficial effect? I know of none.

52. NECESSITY OF VENTILATION—MEANS OF HEATING THE SICK-ROOM—RELATIVE MERITS OF OPEN FIRES, STOVES AND FURNACES.

Next to its intrinsic value, our method gives the patient the great advantage of enjoying *pure fresh air*, either in or out of bed, as it keeps the skin and the whole system in such order as to resist the effects of atmospheric influences better than under a weakening process. And every body knows, or, at least, every body ought to know, that free circulation of fresh air is one of the most important means, in contagious diseases, of preventing the malady from becoming malignant, and of lessening the intensity of the contagion. Although the times are passed, when patients in the heat of fever were almost roasted in their beds, whilst a drink of cooling water was cruelly and stupidly denied them; the temperature of the sick-room is, in general, still kept too high, and not sufficient care is taken to renew the air as frequently, I ought to say as constantly, as necessary for the benefit of the patient. Usually there is no ventilation; very seldom a window is opened, especially in the cold season, when epidemics of scarlatina are most common, and commonly the room is crowded with friends of the patient, who devour the good air, which belongs to him by right, and leave him their exhalations to breathe instead. There is nothing better able to destroy contagious poisons than oxygen and cold; and if we consider that every human being absorbs every minute a volume of air larger than the bulk of its own body, we must understand how necessary it is to keep people away from the sick-room, who are not indispensably necessary to the patient, and to provide for a constant supply of fresh air. But whatever may be the arrangement for that purpose, the patient should not be exposed to a draught. Stoves and fire-places are pretty good ventilators for drawing off the bad air from the room; if you take care not to have too much fire, and to allow a current of pure air to enter at a corresponding place, the top of a window, or a ventilator in the wall opposite the fire-place, there will always be pure air in your sick-room. The air coming from furnaces, which unfortunately have become so general, is good for nothing, especially when taken from the worst place in the house, the cellar or basement. I consider the worst kind of stoves better than the best kind of furnaces; only take care not to heat the stove too much, or to exclude the outer air, which is indispensable to supply the air drawn off by the stove for feeding the fire. The difference between a furnace and a tight stove or fire-place is this: The furnace takes the bad air from the basement or cellar, frequently made still poorer through its passing over red hot iron, which absorbs part of its oxygen, and fills the room with it. The room being filled with poor air, none of the pure air outside will enter it, because there is no vacuum. Thus the bad air introduced into the room, and the bad air created by the persons in it, will be the only supply for the lungs of the patients. But should the furnace take its air from outside the house, as it is the case with some improved kinds, there would still be no ventilation in the sick-room, except there be a fire-place beside the register of the furnace. With the stove or fire-place it is different: The stove continually draws off the lower strata, i. e. the worst part, of the air to feed the fire, whilst pure air will rush in through every crevice of the doors and windows to supply every cubic-inch of air absorbed by the stove. Thus the air in the room is constantly renewed, the bad air being carried off and good air being introduced. However, the openings through which the pure air comes in, must be large enough in proportion to allow a sufficient quantity of air to enter the room to make fully up for the air absorbed by the [Pg 43] stove; for, if not, the air in the room will become thin and poor, and the patient will suffer from want of oxygen. An open fire, from the necessity of its burning brighter and larger to supply sufficient heat, a comparatively large part of which goes off through the chimney, will require a greater supply of air, and consequently larger ventilators or openings for the entrance of the pure air from outside the room. In very cold weather, and in cold climates in general, stoves are preferable to fire-places, the latter producing a draught, and not being able to heat a room thoroughly and equally, causing one side of the persons sitting near them to be almost roasted by the radiant heat in front, whilst their backs are kept cold by the air drawing from the openings in the doors and windows towards the fire to supply the latter. In merely cool weather, and in moderately cold climates, especially in damp places, I would prefer an open fire to a stove. In cold climates stoves are decidedly preferable, especially earthen ones, as they are used in Germany and Russia. Iron stoves must never be heated too much, as the red hot iron will spoil the air of the room, by absorbing the oxygen, as you can easily see by noticing the sparks, which form themselves outside the stove in very hot places.

53. TEMPERATURE OF THE SICK-ROOM.

The *temperature of the sick-room* should not be much above 65° Fahrenheit; in no case should it rise above 70, whilst I do not see the necessity of keeping it below 60, as some hydriatic physicians advise. [31] The patient, in the heat of fever, will think 60° high enough, and rather pleasant; and if others do not like a temperature [Pg 44] as low as that, they may retire. The person necessary for nursing the patient may dress warmly and sit near the fire. Let the sick-room be as large as possible; or open the door and windows of a room connected with it. Towards the close of the disease, after desquamation has begun, the temperature of the room may be kept at 70°, as then the fever and heat have subsided and the delicate skin of the patient requires a comfortable temperature.

54. WATER-DRINKING.

As the patient should have a constant supply of pure air for his lungs, so he should also have *plenty of pure cold water* for his stomach, to allay his thirst and assist in diminishing the heat of fever, and in eliminating the morbid poison from his blood. Though cold, the water for drinking should not be less than 48 or 50° Fahrenheit. Whenever there is ice used for cooling the water, the nurses should be very careful not to let it become colder, than the temperature just indicated, except in typhoid cases, when the stimulating effects of icy cold water and ice may prove beneficial.

55. DIET

I have little to say with regard to *diet*, at least to physicians. During great heat and high fever, the patient should eat little or nothing; but he should drink a good deal. Substantial food must be avoided entirely. When the fever abates, he can take more nourishment, but it should be light. Meat and soup should only be given, when desquamation has fairly begun. Stewed fruit (especially dried apples) will be very agreeable to the patient. In great heat, a glass of lemonade may be given occasionally; however, great care must be taken not to spoil the patient's taste by sweets, or to allow him all sorts of dainties, such as candies, preserves, &c., as it is the habit of weak parents, who like to gratify their [Pg 45] darlings' momentary desires at the expense of their future welfare. In torpid cases, some beef-tea, chicken-broth, and even a little wine with water, will raise the reactive powers of the patient. During convalescence, meat may be permitted to such patients as have been accustomed to eat it, and, in general, the patients may be allowed to gradually resume their former diet (provided it were a healthy one), with some restriction in regard to quantity. In general, under water-treatment, the digestive organs continuing in a tolerably good state, and the functions in better order, we need not be quite so careful with respect to diet, as if the patient were left to himself, or treated after any other method of the drug-system. Let the food be plain, and the patient will scarcely ever eat too much. To stimulate his appetite by constantly asking him whether he would not like this or that, is sheer nonsense; and to satisfy his whims, against our better conviction, is culpable weakness.

From this general outline, I shall now pass to the treatment adapted to the different forms of scarlatina.

56. TREATMENT OF SCARLATINA SIMPLEX, OR SIMPLE SCARLET-FEVER.

Scarlatina simplex, or *simple scarlet-fever* (9), without inflammation of the throat, is generally so mild in its course, that it requires little or no treatment. However, I would not have parents look upon it as "scarcely a disease," as neglect and exposure may bring on bad consequences (7 and 25). If the fever and heat are very moderate, the first days an ablution of the body with cool water (say 70°), twice a day, is sufficient. The patient had better be kept in bed, or, if unwilling to stay there, he should be warmly dressed and move about his room, the temperature of which, in this case, should not be below 70° Fahrenheit, and the windows should be shut, as long as the patient is out of bed.

[Pg 46] When the period of efflorescence, or standing out of the rash, is over, packs ought to be given, to extract the poison completely from the system, and to prevent any sequels, such as anasarca, &c. (25). Should the rash suddenly disappear before the fifth or sixth day, or should it linger in coming out, a long pack will bring it out and remove all danger. The packs, once begun, should be continued, once a day, during and a few days after desquamation. The patient may go out on the tenth or twelfth day warmly dressed, after his pack and bath, and walk for half an hour; sitting down or standing still to talk in the open air is not to be permitted. During, and some time after convalescence, the patient should take a cool bath, or a cold ablution every morning, immediately on rising from bed, and walk after it as soon as he is dressed. In very cold and disagreeable weather, the walk should be taken in the house; but the patient should not sit down, or stand about, before circulation and warmth are completely restored in every part of the body, especially in the feet. I cannot insist too much upon exercise being taken immediately after every bath, as, without it, the bath may do more harm than good, and dressing, with many, will take so much time, that they will take cold before getting their clothes on.

If the patient should take cold, or feel otherwise unwell, during convalescence, the packs must be resorted to again, and continued till he is quite well.

57. TREATMENT OF SCARLATINA ANGINOSA, OR SORE-THROAT SCARLET-FEVER.

In *scarlatina anginosa*, or *sore-throat scarlet-fever*, which is the most common form of the disease (1-7) we have to discriminate, whether

1) the *reaction is mild*, the heat of the body not being much above 100° Fahr. and the pulse full, but not above [Pg 47] 110 to 120, the pain and swelling of the throat moderate, the brain little or not affected; or

2) *violent*, the heat from 106 to 112, the pulse 120 to 150 beats or more, the inflammation of the throat decided and extensive, the brain very much affected; or

3) *torpid*, little or no heat, the pulse quick and weak, the inflammation of the throat undecided, varying, the rash appearing slowly or not at all, and what there appears of a pale, livid color, the patient more or less delirious.

58.—1. TREATMENT OF THE MILD OR ERETHIC FORM OF SCARLATINA ANGINOSA.

The *mild* or *erethic form* of scarlatina anginosa requires about the same treatment as scarlatina simplex. I would, however, for the sake of safety, advise a pack and bath per day, through the whole course of the disease, in the afternoon, when the fever begins to rise; and during the period of eruption, when all the symptoms increase, two and even three packs a day may be required. This depends on the increasing heat and fever, as well as on the condition of the throat. The greater the heat and fever, and the more troublesome the inflammation, the more packs. If the fever and pain increase some time after the pack, in which the patient may stay for an hour or two, the packing must be repeated. The length of the pack depends much on circumstances; as long as the patient feels comfortable and can be kept in it, without too much trouble, he ought to stay. In case the patient cannot be prevailed upon to stay longer than an hour, or if the fever increases soon after the pack, it may be necessary to repeat packing every three or four hours, which is the general practice of several water-physicians in Germany and England.

59. If the patient becomes restless soon after having [Pg 48] been packed, the heat and fever increasing, as may be ascertained from the pulse at the temples and the general appearance of the face, the sheet must be changed, as directed above (46) till the patient becomes quiet and feels more comfortable. In case of repeated changing of sheet, the patient should stay in the last sheet, till he has perspired about half an hour, or longer, before he is taken out to the bath, which should be of about 70°, as in all the mild forms of scarlatina. The length of the bath depends on the heat, and reaction of

the patient, who should be well cooled down all over, before going to bed again or dressing. He ought not to be out of bed for a long time, and only after a bath, as this will protect him from taking cold.

60. The throat should be covered with a wet compress, i. e. a piece of linen four to eightfold, according to its original thickness, dipped in cold water (60°-50°), well wrung out and changed as often as it grows hot. It should be well covered to exclude the air. This compress should be large enough to cover the whole of the throat and part of the chest; it should closely fit to the jaw, and reach as far up as the ear to protect the submaxillary and parotid glands located there.

61. When the period of eruption is over, there is commonly less fever, and the packs and baths may be diminished.

62. Towards the end of the period of efflorescence, when the rash declines, fades, disappears, and the skin begins to peal off, an ablution in the morning of cool water, with which some vinegar *may* be mixed, and a pack and bath in the afternoon, are quite sufficient, except the throat continue troublesome, when a pack should also be given in the morning. The packs, once a day, [Pg 49] should be continued about a week after desquamation. The patient may safely leave the house in a fortnight. I have frequently had my patients out of doors in ten or twelve days, even in winter. [32]

63. This going out so early, in bad weather, is by no means part of the treatment. I mention it only to show the curative and protective power of the latter, and have not the slightest objection to others using a little more caution than I find necessary myself. It is always better, we should keep on the safe side, especially when there is no one near that has sufficient experience in the matter. I can assure my readers upon my word and honor, that though I never kept any of my scarlet-patients longer in-doors than three weeks (except a couple of malignant cases), I have never seen the slightest trouble resulting from my practice.

64. In case of some trouble resulting from early and imprudent exposure, which is about as apt to occur in the house as out of it, a pack or two will usually be [Pg 50] sufficient to restore order again. As long as the patient moves about, warmly dressed, there is no danger of his taking cold after a pack, and provided packing be

continued long enough, and the patient be forbidden to sit down or stand still in cool places, or expose himself to a draught, there is nothing to be apprehended.

65. I have no objection to homœopathic remedies being used at the same time, nor would I consider acids, as mentioned above (39, note), to be objectionable in cases of severe sore throat; but I must caution my readers against the use of any other remedies, especially aperients, except in cases, which I shall mention hereafter (72). In a couple of cases, where I acted as consulting physician, I have observed dropsical symptoms proceeding from laxatives and the early discontinuation of the packs during convalescence. Let the bowels alone as long as you can: there is more danger in irritating them than in a little constipation. As for the rest we have injections, which will do the business without drugs, of which I confess I am no friend, especially in eruptive fevers.

66.—2. TREATMENT OF THE VIOLENT, OR STHENIC FORM OF SCARLATINA ANGINOSA.

The *violent,* or *sthenic form* of scarlatina anginosa becomes dangerous only through the excess of reaction, when the heat is extreme (upwards of 105° Fahrenheit, sometimes 112 to 114), the pulse can scarcely be counted, as it hammers away full and hard in a raging manner, the throat being inflamed and swollen to suffocation, and the patient in a high state of delirium; but it need not frighten the physician or parent acquainted with the use of water. We have the means of subduing that violence without weakening the patient. It is in this form of scarlatina that the greatest mistakes are committed by [Pg 51] physicians unacquainted with the virtues of water, and that our hydriatic method shows itself in all its glory; for where there is an abundance of heat, water cannot only be safely applied, but it is also sure to bring relief. It is in this form of the disease that the cold affusions recommended by Currie and his followers, have shown themselves so beneficial, and that the wet-sheet, used properly and perseveringly, is almost infallible.

67. TEMPERATURE OF THE WATER—DOUBLE SHEET—CHANGING SHEET.

The water for the wet-sheet pack, in this violent form, ought to be cold; in summer it should be iced down to 46-48° Fahr. The sheet ought to be coarse or doubled, in order that it should retain more water, and it should not be wrung out very tight. In a thick wet-sheet the patient will be better cooled than in a thin sheet, and he will be able to stay longer in it before changing. It may be advisable, however, with very young and rather delicate persons, not to double the sheet about the feet, as they might be apt to remain cold, which would send the blood more to the head. But, although the patient will feel easier in the pack for a while, the heat and fever will soon increase again, and, in proportion as the sheet grows warmer, he will become more and more restless, and the changing of the sheet will become indispensable. When the symptoms increase again, in the second pack, the sheet is changed a second time, and so on till the patient perspires and becomes relieved for a couple of hours or longer; which usually happens in the third or fourth sheet. After the first, every following sheet is wrung out tighter and tighter, and the last one may be taken single, or doubled only at its upper end.

[Pg 52] 68. LENGTH OF PACK—PERSPIRATION.

To make quite sure of the reaction, the single sheet may be tried first, except in exceedingly violent cases, and the double sheet may be resorted to, if the single sheet prove inefficient. Or, should there be any doubt, the double sheet may be dipped in water of a higher temperature than that given above, say 55 to 60°. With young and delicate children I prefer this course, especially if they be very excitable, and the shock of very cold water may be expected to be too much for their nerves. In these matters some discrimination should be used: it is always better we should keep on the safe side, and rather give a pack more than frighten the little patients out of their wits. Proceed safely, but firmly and try to obtain your object in the mildest manner possible.

69. Before perspiration comes on, there is a little more excitement for a few minutes (41), which must not induce the friends of the patient to take him out of the pack; only when it continues to increase, instead of the perspiration breaking out and relieving the patient, it will be necessary to change the sheet, another time, as in that case the organism is not fully prepared for perspiration. After the breaking out of the latter, the patient invariably feels easier, and continues so for some time. When the feverish symptoms increase, during perspiration, which can be ascertained by feeling the pulse on the temples and by the thermometer, it is time to remove the patient from the pack, to give him his bath. Half an hour's perspiration is commonly sufficient; if the patient feel easy, however, and can be prevailed upon to stay an hour, or longer, till a good thorough perspiration brings permanent relief, it will be better. It would be unwise to let the patient stay too long and get him in a state of over-excitement; but, on the other hand, parents ought to remember that very [Pg 53] few children *like* to be packed, and that a patient in high fever is a bad judge of his own case. I have always found those children the best patients, who had been brought up in strict obedience to their patients' dictates, before they were sick, and this, as well as the daily habit of taking baths, and the quiet and firm behavior of the physician and friends of the patient under treatment generally remove all difficulty.

70. LENGTH OF BATH.

Although the temperature, in sthenic cases, should be a little lower than in erethic cases, it is not advisable to use the water very cold, as this would cause too strong a reaction, and consequently new excitement. The safer way is to let the temperature of the bath be between 70 and 65°, according to the age and constitution of the patient (the younger and more delicate the patient, the higher the temperature), and to let him stay long enough in the bath to become perfectly cool all over, which can be ascertained by placing the hand or the thermometer under the arm-pits, which usually retain the warmth longest. I understand, in advising such a temperate bath of several minutes, duration, that the patient be hot and the rash standing out full and bright on coming from the pack; or else the bath must be colder and shorter, not exceeding a minute or two.

71. CAUTION.

After the bath, the patient is rubbed dry, and either taken to his bed, or, if he feels well enough, dressed and induced to walk about the room, or placed in a snug corner (not near the fire, however), till he feels tired and wishes to go to bed. During his stay out of bed, the rash ought to be an object of constant attention for his friends; for as soon as it becomes pale, the patient ought to be sent to bed immediately and covered well, or should [Pg 54] then the rash continue to become paler and paler, the pack should be renewed, and the patient kept in bed ever after, till desquamation is over.

72. THE WET COMPRESS.

In bed, a wet compress is put on the throat, and another on the stomach, which, beside the direct influence it has on that organ, acts as a derivative upon the throat and head, and as a diaphoretic upon the skin, assisting in allaying the fever and heat. This compress on the stomach is an excellent remedy with small children and infants in a restless, feverish condition. I often use it, even with infants scarce a week old, and always with perfect success. I wish, mothers could be made to substitute it for paregoric and the like stupefying stuff, to procure their crying infants relief and themselves rest. There is more power in the compress than any one who is not familiar with its use, can imagine. At the same time it has a very good effect on the bowels, which should be kept regular, either with the assistance of tepid injections, or, if they fail to operate, with a moderate dose of castor oil. If possible, however, avoid the irritation of the digestive apparatus through medicines, which are apt to counteract the external applications, whose object is to draw the morbid poison as early and as completely as possible to the skin.

73. HIGHLY INFLAMED THROAT — CROUP.

If the *throat* is in a highly inflamed condition, repeated packing is the surest means of allaying the inflammation and preventing *croup*. Although I have had very bad cases under my hands, I never saw a case of scarlet-croup under water-treatment. All you have to do is, to pack your patient early enough and often enough to keep the inflammation down, to keep a wet compress on his throat and chest, and, in general, treat him as I [Pg 55] have prescribed. The condition of the throat will improve in proportion to your perseverance in packing.

74. NECESSITY OF ALLAYING THE HEAT.

The packs and baths should be continued, even when the patient cannot be prevailed upon to stay long enough in the packs to perspire. The heat of the skin and the general inflammatory condition of the whole organism *must* be allayed, especially, when there is much *delirium*. In that case, the patient ought to be kept long enough in the bath to clear off the head, and care ought to be taken, that he should never stay in the pack to become much excited.

75. THE HALF-BATH — THE SITZ- OR HIP-BATH.

Should the half-bath or shallow-bath (which are technical terms for the bath described above), not be sufficient to relieve the head, the patient must be placed in a *sitz-* or *hip-bath* of 65° to 70° and stay there, with his body covered by a blanket or two, till the head is easy. During and after the sitz-bath, the parts exposed to the water, as well as the lower extremities, should be rubbed repeatedly, to favor the circulation of the blood. The head should be covered with a compress, dipped in cold water and but slightly wrung out, to be changed every time it becomes warm. The time required will vary according to the condition of the patient, from half an hour to one hour and a half. There is no danger of his taking cold, provided the body be covered sufficiently. The room ought not to be too warm, as a hot room will increase the tendency of the blood to the head; 65 to

70° is perfectly warm enough. I would rather have it between 60 and 65.

76. The *sitz-bath* may be taken in a small wash-tub, if there is no proper sitz-bath-tub at hand. It should [Pg 56] be large enough to allow the water to come up to the navel of the patient, and to permit rubbing. Too large a tub would not allow the patient to sit in it comfortably. If there is no tub to fit, a common bathing-tub may be raised on one end, by putting a piece of wood under it, so as to keep the water all in the other end, allowing the feet of the patient to be kept out of the water. This latter practice is more convenient with very small children, with whom, however, the sitz-bath will scarcely be required, a half-bath of sufficient duration being almost always efficient. It is not advisable for persons little acquainted with the use of water as a curative, to let the patient stay very long in the sitz-bath, it being safer to pack the patient again, and to repeat the sitz-bath after the pack, if his delirium is not removed, or not lessened in half an hour or three-quarters of an hour. This alternating with the pack and sitz-bath should be repeated, till the head becomes clear.

77. In excessive heat and continuous delirium, a half-bath may be given, also, every time the packing sheet is changed. The rule is that *we* ought not to yield, but the *symptoms must*; and they will, if the treatment is persevered in. Only go at it with courage and confidence. There is nothing to be apprehended from the treatment: where there is too much heat, there is no danger of a lack of reaction, and consequently no occasion for fears that the rash might be "driven in." A physician afraid of using water freely in violent cases of scarlet-fever, would resemble a fireman afraid of using his engine, for fear of spoiling the house on fire.

78. ACTION OF THE SITZ-BATH EXPLAINED.

The *sitz-bath* acts in a direct manner upon the abdominal organs and the spine, and through the latter on the brain. Indirectly, it helps in removing the [Pg 57] inflammatory and congestive symptoms in the throat and head, by cooling the blood, which circulates through the parts immersed in the water, and by doing so cools also the upper parts of the body, equalizes the temperature, and diminishes the volume of the mass of the blood, thus making its circulation easier, *whilst it has no tendency to impede the action of the skin*. Besides, the abstraction of electricity, by the sitz-bath, should be taken in account of its action. After the sitz-bath, the reaction takes place in those parts which were immersed in the water, thereby making the relief of the upper parts more lasting.

79. RELAXATION OF TREATMENT TOWARDS THE END OF THE THIRD PERIOD—CONTINUATION OF PACKS DURING AND AFTER DESQUAMATION.

When the patient is through the first part of the period of efflorescence the symptoms decrease, and he will be easier. Under the treatment prescribed, the time when the excitement is highest, is much abridged, and usually the treatment can be relaxed in less than twenty-four hours. When the patient is easier, the treatment may be given as in the milder form of scarlatina anginosa, with due regard to the state of the throat. In proportion as the heat abates, the packs should not be repeated so often, the sheet not changed; the patient should stay longer in the packs, and the baths should be shorter. The sitz-bath would then be out of season. The packing should be repeated whenever the symptoms increase again; but even if they should not, one pack and bath a day are necessary.

80. During and after desquamation, the treatment should be continued as indicated in milder cases, except the throat continue troublesome, when more packs should be used. If the throat is well, the patient may leave his room by the sixteenth day, under the precautions given above.

[Pg 58] 81.—3. TREATMENT OF TORPID FORMS OF SCARLATINA—DIFFERENCE IN THE TREATMENT POINTED OUT.

When the *reaction* is *torpid*, the pulse small, weak, quick, the skin dry, the rash slow to appear, and when it appears in small, pale, livid spots, instead of bright scarlet patches (16-25); the treatment ought to be calculated to produce a short, but powerful, stimulus upon the surface of the body, after which a long pack should assist the organism in producing a slow, continuous and increasing reaction. If in violent reaction a repetition of short packs and long cooling baths is indicated,—in torpid reaction, cold and short tonic baths or affusions and long packs are required, in proportion to the degree of the reactive power of the patient. Therefore the packing sheet should be very cold, but thin and well wrung out, so as to make a strong, but transitory, impression, soon overcome by the reaction it calls forth, upon which all our success depends. The patient stays in the pack till he becomes quite warm and tired. Perspiration is seldom produced; if it is, it may be considered a favorable symptom. I have had patients stay in the pack for four, five, six and seven hours, and almost always, when I took them out, their skin was covered with eruption. The only phenomenon, which should induce the physician to relieve the patient of the pack before he becomes perfectly warm, is increased delirium, which in torpid reaction, indicates a tendency to a typhoid character of the disease, when the warm and moist atmosphere of the long pack would be more favorable to the disease than to the patient, by weakening the nerves still more. In that case, a long half-or sitz-bath is required, the former, under constant rubbing, from 15 to 20 minutes, the latter from 30 to 40 minutes; the temperature of either from 65° to 70°.

[Pg 59] 82. LENGTH OF PACK.

Usually it is time for the patient to come out from his pack, when the pulse becomes fuller and stronger, the face begins to flush and the head to be affected. Frequently he sleeps till awakened by the increasing heat. A drink of cold water will quiet him for a while, which may be administered by means of a glass tube (julep-tube), in order not to disarrange the pack by lifting him up. As long as the head is not affected, there is no danger of his staying too long. The longer he can stay, the surer the eruption will appear.

83. COLD AFFUSIONS AND RUBBING.

After the pack, the patient is placed in an empty bathing or washtub, and cold water (of 65°-60° Fahr., only with very young and delicate children a little higher, with adults rather lower) is thrown over him in quick succession by means of a dipper, whilst he is well rubbed all over his body, especially the extremities. Not too much water should be poured over the head; however, the head should be always wetted first. This process should not last longer than a minute or two, except the patient continue very warm during it, in which case it should be prolonged, as the perfect cooling of the body is necessary to prevent the fever from coming on soon after and the patient continuing weak. After the bath, he should be rubbed dry, first with the bare hands of the attendants, and then with a dry sheet, and put to bed again, or, if he feel inclined to stay up, dressed warmly and be induced to walk about as long as he can.

84. ICE-WATER AND SNOW-BATH IN MALIGNANT CASES.

If no rash appear during the first pack, which will scarcely fail, the proceeding should be repeated, and the patient stay longer in the pack than the first time. In very bad cases, when the patient fails at once under the [Pg 60] action of the poison (malignant scarlet-fever) iced water or snow may be resorted too. I know several instances of patients, having been given up by their physicians, reviving again under the influence of a snow-bath, which produced a healthy reaction, when nothing else was of avail. I have never had occasion myself to resort to such extremes, cold water having always answered my purposes; but I would not hesitate a minute to use snow and ice in a case where I could think it useful and necessary. Such proceedings *look* cruel; but it *is* decidedly more cruel to let the patient's life be destroyed from want of timely assistance. I distinctly remember a case, which occurred in Cassel, when the physician objected to "tormenting the poor boy," and wanted the father to "let him die in peace." But the father, [33] who had some knowledge of, and a great deal of confidence in hydriatics, put the little patient, a boy of 8 or 9 years, into a bathing-tub filled for the greater part with snow, covered him over with the cold material, and left him there till he became conscious; then he was rubbed all over, placed in a dry pack (without a sheet), and left to perspire, which ensued and brought out the rash. The patient was out of danger in four hours' time, and Dr. S., on calling again in the evening, was quite astounded at seeing him alive, out of bed, and covered with a tolerably bright eruption.

85. WINE AND WATER, IF NO REACTION CAN BE OBTAINED.

Should the patient remain cold in his pack for longer than an hour,—a case, which will seldom occur,—a little wine and water may be given him to assist the organism in producing a reaction; and, in case of need, the dose may be repeated once or twice in intervals of half an hour. The quantity should be adapted to the age and [Pg 61] constitution of the patient, and by no means sufficient to affect the head. Instead of water, it may also be mixed with warm broth or tea, or hot water and sugar, to make it agreeable to the little patient.

86. ABLUTIONS AND RUBBING WITH ICED WATER OR SNOW.

In a few very obstinate cases, when no rash would appear after two or three long packs, I have succeeded by washing the patient with ice-water or snow, rubbing him dry with my bare hands, and then packing him in a dry blanket. After staying there for several hours, more or less eruption always appeared.

87. WET COMPRESS.

The wet compress on the throat in torpid cases should not be changed often, but left till it becomes almost dry. Should the feet of the patient be cold, a bottle filled with hot water and wrapped in a piece of blanket or a sheet should be placed near them, either within the pack, or out of it, when the patient is lying in bed. The feet should always be kept warm.

88. VENTILATION ALL-IMPORTANT.

If the circulation of air is necessary in any other form of scarlet-fever, it is all-important in torpid reaction, especially when it inclines to a typhoid type. We should never forget that it is the oxygen of the air that nourishes the process of combustion going on in every living body, and that in the same manner as no fire can burn bright without a sufficient supply of air, the combustion within the patient will be slower in proportion as there is less pure air in the sick-room, and consequently his reaction will be weaker, and *vice versa*. A sick-room, filled with a number of people, and with a large fire in it, or fed with the corrupted air of a furnace, without the access of pure air, will always prove a dangerous place [Pg 62] for a patient in torpid fever, the fire and every living soul in it absorbing the oxygen indispensable to his recovery. And if the case become typhoid, there is little hope of saving the patient's life without plenty of pure air.

89. CONTINUATION OF PACKS—CONVALESCENCE.

Whether the eruption appear or not, the packs should be continued during the whole course of the disorder, and as long as the throat continues troublesome; and one pack and bath a day should be given during some ten or twelve days, after every symptom has disappeared. The patient, during convalescence should not go out, except after his bath and in fine sunny weather, till he feels quite well. However, he should not be kept unnecessarily too long indoors either, as exercise in the open air will assist him in regaining his strength. If the weather is clear and bright, the low temperature of the air need not be minded. I never saw any one take cold after a pack and bath that walked out warmly dressed in clear and cold weather.

90. MINERAL ACIDS, IN CASE OF SEVERE SORE-THROAT.

In case the throat be very troublesome, there cannot be any objection to using the mineral acid, as I have indicated above (35), except homœopathic remedies should be thought preferable and found to afford sufficient relief. Some good may, and no harm can be done by either.

91. PUTRID SYMPTOMS—GARGLE—SOLUTION OF CHLORIDE OF SODA—DRINK: CHLORATE OF POTASS—LIQUOR CALCII-CHLORIDI.

Should *putrid symptoms* make their appearance (21), I would strongly advise the acid in full and repeated doses, as well as the frequent repetition of the packs. In [Pg 63] putrid cases, not only the syrup, but also the gargle will do good service. Gargling is so much the more advisable as the putrid matter should be frequently removed. If nothing else can be had, pure water or water and vinegar may be used. The temperature of the gargle should be about 70°-75° Fahrenheit. For the same purpose, the *aqua chlorina*, and the *chloride of soda* have been strongly recommended. [34] A few drops of the solution may be used, also, on the compress outside.

92. TREATMENT OF AFFECTIONS OF THE NERVOUS CENTRES.

In affections of the nervous centres, the *brain*, the *cerebellum*, and the *spine* (see 17-19), the danger which [Pg 64] threatens the patient's life is principally averted by the sitz-bath. The nervous system needs support, and the circulation must be regulated. In every case where the packs do not relieve the symptoms in the head and spine, the sitz-bath is probably the only remedy to remove the danger. It should be about 70°, and the patient should stay in it till relieved, which will probably be in half an hour or there about. After the sitz-bath, if the patient feels quite easy and inclined to sleep, he may be put to bed; if he continues restless and still complains of pain, he should be put in a wet pack of about 65°. There he should stay till he complains of more pain, when he should take his bath and repeat the sitz-bath. Thus he should alternate till he becomes entirely relieved.

93. SITZ-BATH, ANCHOR OF SAFETY.

If there be much delirium, the sitz-bath may be required longer, and the pack shorter, as indicated above (81). In all such cases the packs and sitz-baths, alternately, ought to be continued, till the nervous symptoms disappear altogether, and should they make their appearance again, the treatment must be resumed without delay.

94. I repeat that in such cases, the sitz-bath is the only anchor of safety I know of. I have tried to remove these dangerous symptoms by packs, affusions, baths, but almost always in vain; whilst the sitz-bath has never failed to insure success. As I am the only writer on hydriatic treatment of scarlatina (as far as I know), who mentions the virtue of the sitz-bath in those cases, and as I am probably the first who ventured to use it, with one of my own children, in 1836, when all seemed to fail, I shall corroborate my advice by a couple of cases.

[Pg 65] 95. CASES.

During an epidemic of scarlatina in 1836 two of my children were attacked by the disease, a boy of about eight, and another of five years, the younger one two days after the older one. I ordered them to be packed, and all seemed to go well, when, during my absence from the city (of Freiberg) a medical friend, who called, persuaded my wife to desist from continuing the hydriatic treatment, and use some remedies of his instead. On my return, I found the elder boy (the other began only to show some slight symptoms) in a very bad state: the cerebellum and spine were distinctly affected by the contagious poison; the patient complained of insupportable pain in the back of his head, the spine and all over his body, so that no one dared to touch him. The fact of the packs having been discontinued during twenty-four hours being concealed from me, and the boy being subject to herpes and inclined to scrofula, I began to fear that the treatment would not be applicable in such cases, and became really alarmed about my child. I was then almost a novice in Priessnitz's practice, at least in the treatment of acute diseases, which seldom occurred at Græfenberg, and, had I had more confidence in blood-letting and drugs, I would probably have resorted to them. For a while I was doubtful about the course I should pursue, when Dr. B., my medical friend, made his appearance and I learned what had happened during my absence. Instead, however, of giving way to his earnest solicitations to rely on the old practice, I at once became encouraged by his confession, and declared I would persevere in my own practice, which was quite new to him, and in which no physician of the place as yet believed. He assured me, from the symptoms, that the boy could not live twenty-four hours, unless he be bled, and that even then he would not answer for his life. Having lost six children before under allopathic treatment, and [Pg 66] having never had much confidence in drugs during the time I had been connected myself with the practice, I firmly refused to allow either bleeding or drugging, and expressed my resolution to see what water could do, resigning myself to the possibility of a bad issue of the case. I need scarcely assure my readers, that my feelings were far from agreeable, and that my resolution required all the reminiscence of the bad success of allopathic treatment of former cases in my family, and the confidence I had in Priessnitz and his system, to support it. I tried the pack again, which did little or no good. Judging from the effects of the sitz-bath in cases of affection of the brain during continued fevers, that it might be of service also in the present case (Priessnitz's directions did not go so far, nor had I treated a similar case since my return from Græfenberg), I put my boy with great care into a sitz-bath of 70° F. and left him there for a little over half an hour, when he felt greatly relieved. He was taken to his bed and allowed to become warm, when he began to complain again. I then packed him, seemingly without much effect; therefore the sitz-bath was repeated and proved quite successful. I then packed the patient immediately after the sitz-bath and left him two hours in the pack, where he slept almost all the time. When he awoke, he complained again of pain in his head, which partly yielded to the half-bath. About three hours after the bath, he complained more of the pain in his head and spine, and I repeated the sitz-bath and the pack. He slept in the pack for about three hours, and when I took him out, he was covered with red spots. Feeling pretty well, he was dressed and permitted to stay up. In the forenoon, my friend called to see whether our patient were still living, and could hardly believe his own eyes when, on cautiously putting his head in at the door, he saw the boy walking up and down the room to warm his feet. In the afternoon, the [Pg 67] pain returned and the rash faded. I repeated the pack, and the pain not yielding entirely, I gave him one more sitz-bath in the evening and a pack after it, in which he stayed asleep almost all the time, nearly four hours, upon which the rash stood out finely and never disappeared until desquamation set in. I managed to keep him in bed after the relapse mentioned, till desquamation was over. I need scarcely say that I continued to pack him (twice a day) till after desquamation, when the packs were given once a day for about a week longer. On the seventeenth day (which was the fifteenth with the younger boy, who had the fever in a very mild form, and was treated accordingly) the two scarlet-convalescents were seen playing in the street, throwing snowballs at each other; a fact, which increased not a little the sensation caused by this miraculous cure. Although my friend was not converted to the new method, this case had a very decided encouraging influence upon myself, and, I am convinced, became the means of salvation for many hundred lives afterwards, treated partly by myself directly, partly by other physicians, or the parents of the patients, after my prescriptions. I felt the importance of my success in this difficult case of scarlatina, and warmly thanked Providence for having assisted me in saving my child for the benefit of many others. [35]

96. The circumstance that, at the same time my two boys were taken sick with scarlatina, a servant of mine became afflicted with *small-pox*, my daughter with *varioloids*, and my mother and wife with *influenza*, [Pg 68] afforded me an ample opportunity of trying the effects of the water-cure and my own courage and skill in the new method. The servant was cured, chiefly by long packs, in

twelve days, so that she was able to resume her household duties, and though she had been covered with pocks all over, not the slightest mark remained on her body; my little girl was out of doors in a fortnight, and a few days were sufficient to rid the ladies of influenza. The complete success I had in the treatment of all these cases, contributed not a little to encourage me to employ the method upon others, with whom I have ever since been equally successful, with one single exception, which I shall mention hereafter.

97. One of the last cases of affection of the brain in torpid scarlatina I treated, was that of a scrofulous little boy of six years, from Williamsburgh, N. Y., who was at my establishment, with his mother and sisters, taking treatment for scrofulous ulceration of the parotid glands, and other symptoms of that dangerous disease. The reaction was torpid, and the brain became affected almost from the commencement. There was a little rash coming out, but in small dark purple spots, looking much more like measles than scarletfever. The delirium increased during the period of efflorescence, instead of giving way. The spine evidently sympathized in the suffering of the brain and cerebellum. Homœopathic remedies, which were earnestly asked for by the mother, had no effect whatever; acids only produced a slight relief of the inflammation of the throat; the packs increased the symptoms in the head and spine. The appearance of the tongue, the peculiar kind of delirium, the small quick pulse, &c. showed, that the case was going to take a typhoid turn; when I ordered a sitz-bath, which almost immediately relieved the head and improved the pulse, I then, proceeded in about the same [Pg 69] manner as described above in my son's case, with the difference, that I allowed longer intervals. The patient, according to the severity of the symptoms, took one or two packs a day, and the same number of sitz-baths, had wet compresses on his ears and throat, and was kept in bed with very few exceptions, when the nurse would take him on her knees, wrapt in a blanket. The good effect of the sitz-bath was so obvious, that the child's father, who had been informed by telegraph of the critical condition of his son, asked himself for a repetition of it, when he found that neither medicines nor packs produced the slightest change. The child always became quiet and slept after the bath. Not only was his life saved, but he also escaped all the dreaded consequences of the disease. I

am confident, that under any other kind of treatment, he would have lost his life, or at least he would have lost his hearing. But, far from increasing, the affection of his ears was rather improved when he left, and his general health a great deal better than when he was first placed under my care. I had a great deal of trouble with that little patient, not only because he did not allow me a night's rest for a week, and the case produced quite an estampeda in the establishment, [36] but [Pg 70] also, and chiefly, because of the interference of a half-bred Irish woman, who had brought him up, and who, on account of the mother's bad health, acted in the double quality of a nurse and a governess towards the children. This woman, being averse to the treatment and the place, which gave her little pleasure, and to the rules of which she would not submit, procured all sort of dainties and excited the child by her foolish remonstrances against any application I found necessary, making at the same time an unfavorable impression on the simple minds of the family, by telling lies and tales, thereby not only placing difficulties in my way, in a case which was difficult in itself, but even preventing the parents from acknowledging by one word of thanks the sacrifices of time and health I had cheerfully made. What a blessing it would be for physicians and patients, could unnecessary and unreasonable people be kept away from persons afflicted with painful and dangerous diseases! —

[Pg 71] 98. IMPOSSIBILITY OF ANSWERING FOR THE ISSUE OF EVERY TYPHOID CASE.

Although a *typhoid character* of scarlatina will rarely set in, when the patient has been subject to the packs from the beginning of the disease, there will be cases when water-treatment can neither prevent such an event or even save the life of the patient afflicted by scarlet-fever. There will be a case, *now and then*, to baffle any mode of treatment, and the physician must not be blamed for losing a patient of scarlatina occasionally, but it is not necessary that people should continue to die of this disease in such numbers, as they have been destroyed till now.

99. Any case, where typhoid symptoms set in (16-25), is dangerous, and the physician and his mode of treatment deserve commendation, if the patient is saved by it; and it is in such cases, also, that the hydriatic physician requires the most skill, experience and courage.

100. IS WATER APPLICABLE IN ALL TYPHOID CASES?

The question has been raised, whether in typhoid cases, and in cases of torpid reaction in general, water is at all applicable? I can answer the question only in the affirmative; but I must add, that the treatment of such cases requires more than confidence and courage: it requires a nice discrimination to know the exact moment, when water may be applied, what should be its temperature, how long the bath should last, what kind of baths should be given, whether the pack will be of service, &c.

101. RULES FOR THE APPLICATION OF WATER IN TYPHOID CASES.

As a general rule, in typhoid cases, bathing should form one of the principal features of the treatment; i. e. the patient should have more baths than packs in proportion to the treatment of other cases.

[Pg 72] 102. The temperature of the baths should be in proportion to the reactive power of the body; i. e. the longer the patient has been sick, and the weaker he is, the higher should be the temperature of the water, but never so high as to have rather a weakening than a strengthening effect upon the nervous system. The highest temperature which may be used should not exceed 75° F.

103. When the delirium is active, the patient restless, almost raging, the water should be used colder; when the delirium is more passive, the patient weak, muttering, the water should be warmer: in the former case, the water may be between 50 and 60°, in the latter, between 60 and 70°.

104. When the skin is hot and dry, a wet-sheet pack will produce relief, and assist in bringing out the rash. After the pack, a half-bath should be given, the duration of which must be regulated by the condition of the brain. If the delirium continues, the bath should be prolonged.

105. The patient should not leave the bath before his head is clearer. It may be necessary for the patient to stay in the bath for more than half an hour.

106. In a low condition, with passive delirium, the packs should not be continued very long, as they will be apt to increase the bad condition of the brain. In that case they should be used only to prepare the body for the bath following it.

107. When the skin is cool and moist, neither a bath nor a pack is indicated. When the skin is rather cool and dry, an affusion of cold water and frictions with the bare hands should be used, and the patient packed afterwards in a dry blanket, to assist in producing a [Pg 73] reaction. In such cases I have found very cold water to be of more service than water of a warmer temperature. When the patient has not been too much weakened already, a rash is likely to be produced by the proceeding, and in consequence of repeated baths, the nervous system to be relieved and a healthier reaction to be obtained.

108. Should putrid symptoms appear, I would advise the use of mineral acids and chloride of lime, in addition to hydriatic treatment.

109. In no case would I advise a hydriatic practitioner to overdo, either in regard to the temperature or to the quantity of the baths. The state of the brain and of the skin should always guide him. The increase of delirium will require a bath, and the dryness and heat of the skin a pack. If both symptoms exist, the bath is to be preferred, as the condition of the nervous system should always command the principal attention of the physician. When the nervous system is supported, the whole of the organism is, and the condition of the skin usually improves with the former.

110. ILLUSTRATIONS.

I shall give a couple of illustrations:

In the winter of 1845-46, during an epidemic, which ravaged the city of Dresden and the neighboring villages, I was called to see a child, belonging to a tradesman, blessed with a large family, but without sufficient means to support them. I found the whole family crammed together in a room of moderate size, the patient lying in a bed near the window. There was a large fire in a sheet-iron stove, upon which the mother was preparing the scanty dinner of the family. The air was filled with the exhalations of the living, beside the smell from the [Pg 74] potatoes and sourkrout, which was undergoing the cooking process, the sundry boots and shoes lying around or being under repair in the hands of the father, and a few pieces of linen hanging behind the stove for the purpose of drying. In an adjoining alcove lay the body of a little boy, who had expired the day before, a victim of scarlet-fever.

I found the patient, a fair-haired little girl of about eight years, in a state of sopor, which had lasted a day and a half; there had been delirium for two or three days, during which time the child had never had a clear moment. There was a purple rash all over the body. The temperature of the body I found 112 F., on placing my pocket-thermometer under the pit of the arm; the pulse was small, but exceedingly quick. There was considerable inflammation of the throat and swelling of the face; the breath was very bad. There was a blister on the throat and a mustard plaster on each of the soles of the feet.

I sent for a large wash-tub and water, which I mixed with some warm water, so as to make it about 65°. I had the child undressed, and placed in the empty tub, after removing the blister and mustard; then I poured the water slowly over her head, shoulders and the rest of the body. The second pail brought her to consciousness, but only for a moment. As the delirium returned, I continued to pour water over her; till the tub was filled about nine inches, when I used the water from the bath. In fifteen minutes, I found the heat of the body diminished about five degrees. Soon after, the child became conscious, and its mind cleared off more and more, as she continued in the bath. In thirty minutes, the heat was 103, and the pulse, which first could not be counted, 135, when I removed her from the bath and put her in a wet-sheet pack, where she fell asleep. The pulse continuing slower, coming down to 126, and the heat not increasing, [Pg 75] I left her in the pack for an hour and three quarters, when I observed an increase of heat, a quickening of the pulse and a return of delirium.

The water of the first bath still standing in the room, but having become warmer, and it being found troublesome to carry much water up-stairs to a fifth story; I sent for a pail more of fresh water, lowering the temperature of the bath to 71°, and, placing the child in the bath, threw water over it, as I had done before. This time the bath produced a beneficial effect much sooner, and I removed the patient from it in about twelve minutes. The heat of the body had gone down to 101, the pulse was 118, and the patient was perfectly conscious, complaining a good deal of her throat. I placed a wet compress on the throat and chest and had her put to bed, but ordered the bed to be removed further from the window, and the latter partly to be kept open. I need scarcely say, that I had opened it soon after entering the room.

When I returned in about five hours, I found the patient covered with a thick feather-bed, the window closed, the air of the room as bad as before; the patient was delirious, the heat 110, the pulse upwards of 150.

I repeated the bath as before, but continued only twenty minutes; then I packed her again, placed a wet compress on her head, opened the window entirely, and left, promising to be back in an hour.

This time, on my return, I found the window open, the air better, the child conscious in her pack. I left her a quarter of an hour longer; then placed her in a bath of fresh water, of 70°, kept her there five minutes, and put her back to bed. It being late in the evening, I recommended changing the compress on the throat and placing another on the stomach, and in case of renewed delirium, a cold compress on the head, to be changed frequently.

When I called in the morning, I found the patient again in delirium, the heat 110°, the pulse 140.

The bath was repeated for twenty-five minutes, when the heat went down to 100°, and the pulse to 120. The patient being conscious, I had her packed again and left her about two hours in the pack. When I returned, I found her head almost clear; the bath of 70° for ten minutes brightened her very much. Her throat continued very troublesome, one of the submaxillary glands was very much swollen, and broke afterwards, on the fifth day of my treatment, discharging fetid matter. Also the parotid gland on the same side became seriously affected, swoll considerably and looked as if the ear might be endangered. The patient developing heat enough, I used nothing but wet compresses, and water and vinegar for a gargle.

The heat and delirium returning, the patient was bathed and packed twice more the same day; the pack lasting only an hour to an hour and a quarter. The night was pretty good; there was little delirium.

The third day, the patient was packed twice, and had four baths, and the bowels being costive, an injection of tepid water in the evening.

The fourth day, the rash having disappeared, and the heat being down to 98, whilst the pulse continued weak and quick, and the patient still had some delirium, I gave her a pack in the forenoon, without a bath previous, of an hour and a half, and a short bath after it; and in the afternoon, the patient having more delirium, the half-bath of 70° was repeated, and the patient kept in it for twenty minutes.

On the fifth day the ulcerating gland burst outside and the parotid gland became relieved. Pack and baths as the day before. In the evening the patient complaining of pain in the bowels, a sitz-bath of 70° for twenty minutes was administered, and an injection after it, which relieved her.

The rest of the time, one pack and bath in the morning, and a bath in the afternoon were deemed sufficient. On the eighteenth day of my treatment the patient left the house for the first time, and continued improving from day to day, the packs being continued for about two weeks longer on account of the broken gland, which continued to discharge. I tried to persuade the parents to continue the packs till the gland was healed, but they found it too much trouble.

The patient drank a good deal of water during the whole of the treatment, ate very little and only light food, principally water-soup or panada, and gruel, and kept in bed almost entirely the first ten or twelve days. Her deceased little brother had the same symptoms, and I am confident, she would have followed him, had she not come under hydriatic treatment.

111. A later case, to which I have alluded before, was the following: The driver of a lady, who was under my care in Florence, attending to one of the lady's maids, who was sick with typhoid scarlatina, was taken ill. Like most uneducated people, he could not understand how water could do any good for diseases, and went to the village-store to buy some patent medicine, which he took. The remedy producing no good effect, he bought some other medicine—purgative pills, as I understood—and took it. Some friends of the village, which, like other villages, especially in America, was full of doctors—brought him nostrums and popular remedies, which he took for some days, till he could not leave the bed any more, delirium set in, and I was at last applied for. I found him with all the symptoms of typhus, and scarcely any of scarlatina, except the tongue, which seemed to struggle between a typhoid and scarlatinous appearance, but soon took all the form and color of the former. There was no rash, not much of a sore-throat, but constant delirium and rapid sinking of the strength of the patient.

[Pg 78] Under these circumstances, I believed I must treat him more for typhus than for scarlatina, and used cold baths; in which course I was encouraged by the fine reaction ensuing after every bath, and the slight clearing off of his mind for a few minutes. Internally, I used the muriatic-acid in the forms mentioned above (39), and the solution of chloride of lime, which was also used for a wash and sprinkled about the room. In order to draw the eruption towards the skin—provided there be any of the scarlatinous poison in his system,—I tried a few packs, but without avail. He grew weaker and weaker, though his skin continued to become red after every bath, and on the sixth day early in the morning, when we were about changing his linen, and I was holding him sitting up in bed, he expired in my arms. This is the only case of scarlet-fever, I lost under hydriatic treatment; and it is yet doubtful whether it can be considered as belonging to that disease. I have always considered it, and continue to do so now, a case of typhus, partly communicated by the typhoid exhalations of the other servant, and partly created in his own body, as he complained for more than a fortnight before, of nervous and feverish symptoms, which indicated a serious disease threatening him. The contagion of scarlatina may have made the case more dangerous by complicating it; but, be this as it may, it is certain that the symptoms were such from the beginning that a cure must have appeared most improbable at first sight to any physician of any school; and if there was a possibility of saving his life, it could only be done by the course I took; a course which had proved successful in several cases of typhus I had treated before, and which looked about as bad, and even worse than that of poor William McNought.

112. The young woman, who apparently communicated the typhoid contagion to William, was in quite as [Pg 79] critical a condition as her fellow-servant; and for a while I doubted of her recovery. She continued delirious for more than a fortnight, and there were distinct putrid symptoms, her throat and glands ulcerating, and breaking in two places outside. For longer than a week she had not a lucid moment, became extenuated and powerless. We had to lift her into the baths and out; involuntary discharges from the bowels and the bladder took place; petechiæ appeared, and every thing indicated a steady decay. Neither acids nor chloride of lime seemed to have any effect; the only thing, which revived her, was the tepid half-bath, of 70°, which she took twice a day for about twenty minutes. She was usually carried into the bath-room near by, and was commonly able to walk back assisted by the nurses. She took a pack occasionally for an hour or an hour and a half, as long as a few spots of the rash made their appearance. Her skin peeled off but imperfectly (there was not an appearance of desquamation on the driver's person, although he died about the tenth day after the disease had manifested itself). The patient not producing much heat, I used a poultice of hemlock-leaves and bran on her glands, the gargle of muriatic-acid, and ablutions of water and vinegar externally, when the skin was not prepared for a bath. Although of a weak,

scrofulous habit, and having always been sickly, not only her life was saved, but her health became afterwards stronger, and her looks much better than they ever were before. The gland kept discharging for three or four months longer, and I have no doubt, to her great benefit.

With this patient, I never found the heat to exceed 100° Fahr. and the delirium never had a very active character. For the greater part of the time, her skin was more cool than warm, and sometimes even clammy.

FOOTNOTES:

[7] Elements of Medicine, Vol. I. London, 1836.

[8] J. Armstrong, Practical Illustrations of the scarlet-fever, measles, &c. London, 1818.

[9] W. Withering. An account of the scarlet-fever, &c. London, 1779.

[10] Hamilton, in Edinburgh Journal.

[11] F. Jahn, in Hufeland's Journal, 1829.

[12] J. Wendt, das Wesen, die Bedeutung und ærztl. Behandl. des Scharlachs. Breslau, 1819.

[13] F. A. G. Berndt, D. Scharlachepidemie im Küstriner Kreise, 1817-19, &c. Berlin, 1820. — The same, Bemerk. über das Scharlachfieber, &c. Greifswalde, 1827.

[14] Peart, Practical informations on malignant scarlet-fever and sore-throat, in which a new mode of treatment is freely communicated. London, 1802.

[15] J. B. Brown, On scarlatina, and its successful treatment by the Acidum-aceticum-dilutum of the Pharmacopæia. London, 1846.

[16] The forms in which I have given this acid are the following:

Take three ounces of raspberry syrup and fifteen drops of muriatic acid. Rub the whole of the acid with two or three spoonfuls of syrup in a porcelain mortar (or, if there is none, in a soup-plate with the foot of a wine-glass, or a tumbler) for a minute or two; then add some more of the syrup and rub again, and thus continue till the acid is well divided and mixed up with the syrup. Of this mixture give the patient a teaspoonful every hour or two, or oftener, according to the symptoms.

An other form for a gargle is this:

Take a cup of coarse pearl-barley (or of rice), roast it till yellow; then boil it with one quart of water for ten minutes; add one teaspoonful of muriatic-acid, and four or six tablespoonfuls of honey; mix it well and use it for a gargle, tepid. The decoction should be passed through some linen, or a sieve, before the acid and honey are added, to keep back the barley or rice-grains.

The syrup should be used for inflammation of the tonsils; the gargle for inflammation of the fauces or pharynx.

[17] Schnitzlein, das Scharlachfieber, seine Geschichte, Erkenntniss und Heilung: München, 1851.

[18] Schneemann, die sichere Heilung der Scharlachkrankheit durch eine neue, völlig gefahrlose Heilmethode. Hannover, 1848.

[19] Lindsley, Boston Med. and Surg. Journal, May, 1850.

[20] C. A. W. Richter, das Wasserbuch. Berlin, 1856.

[21] Berend, Oppenheimer Zeitschrift. April, 1848.

[22] Hauner, Deutsche Klinik, 1850, No. 41.

[23] Hufeland, Hedenus, Burdach, Berndt, Cramer, Maclure, Féron, &c.

[24] Lehmann, Harnier, Wagner, Vogel, Steimmig, Schwartze, Cock, Pfaff, Baumgärtner, Belitz, &c.

[25] Currie, on the effects of cold and tepid water. London.

[26] Kolbany, Beobacht. über den Nutzen des lauen und kalten Wassers im Scharlachf. Pressburg, 1808.

[27] Reuss, d. Wesen der Exantheme. Nürnberg, 1818. Vol. III.

[28] A. Edler von Fröhlichsthal, Abhandl. über d. kräftige, sichere und schnelle Wirkung der Uebergiessungen &c. im Faul-, Nerven-, Gallen-, Brenn- und Scharlachfieber. Wien, 1842.

[29] L. Hesse, in Rust's Magaz. Vol. XXVII. 1.

[30] R. Steimmig, Erfahr. und Betracht. über d. Scharlachfieber und seine Behandl. Karler., 1828.

[31] P. ex. Reich, who kept the sick-room quite cold, and made his scarlet-patients walk out in any weather; he assures us that he cured his patients in five days, an interesting fact, for the correctness of which, however, the Doctor alone is responsible.

[32] A visit at my establishment of a gentleman, a short time ago, whom I treated for scarlatina anginosa in the city of New-York in February, 1851, reminds me of the sensation caused among his friends by our walking out together on the tenth day in a snow-storm, to take dinner at a restaurant's, where we consumed a partridge and sundry other articles, after which we took a further walk of half an hour. Some physicians of my acquaintance told me "I was killing the man," to which I replied, I would let them know, when he was dead. However, he never experienced the slightest inconvenience from his early exposure; on the contrary, he felt bright and strong on coming home, and has been in pretty good health ever since. He saved, last year, the life of a nephew, who had been given up, by packing him, in scarlet-fever, whilst two of the patient's sisters were allowed to die soon after—unpacked!—Their uncle had been compelled to leave the place of their residence, and the parents had neither courage nor confidence in the water-cure to repeat the process, though their son—whom I saw a few weeks afterwards in vigorous health,—had been saved by it. They had more confidence in drugs which had done nothing for him.

[33] Mr. Rossteuscher, who became afterwards proprietor of a water-cure-establishment near Cassel.

[34] "And something may be done by way of gargles, to correct the state of the throat, and to prevent the distressing and perilous consequences, which would otherwise be likely to flow from it. A weak solution of the chloride of soda may be employed for this purpose; and if the disease occur in a child that is not able to gargle, this solution may be injected into the nostrils and against the fauces, by means of a syringe or elastic bottle. The effect of this application is sometimes most encouraging. A quantity of offensive sloughy matter is brought away; the acid discharge is rendered harmless; the running from the nose and diarrhœa cease, &c."

"From several distinct and highly respectable sources, *chlorine* itself has been strongly pressed upon my notice, as a most valuable remedy in the severest forms of scarlet-fever." Watson, Principles and Practice of Physic.

Dr. Watson also recommends a *drink*, prepared of a drachm of *chlorate of potass* to a pint of water, and has found great improvement from the use of a pint to a pint and a half of this solution daily.

Brown gives his scarlet-patients the pure *liquor calcii chloridi*, or the *aqua oxymuriatica* in quantities of one teaspoonful every two or three hours and considers this remedy as almost a specific. A solution of the same remedy may be used as a gargle, and also as a wash; and if used internally, I would rather recommend it in preference to the pure liquor, in the hands of persons not used to medical practice. In putrid cases, also the packing sheet may be dipped in a thin solution of chloride. — From an aversion to drugs — very natural in a hydriatic physician — I have never tried medicated sheets, getting along very nicely without them, but I think they must have sufficient virtue to recommend themselves to physicians and parents, who would like to try them.

[35] Captain Claridge, who communicated the above case to the English, and by reprint also to the American public, erroneously reported it a case of *measles*. How he could have made the mistake, I do not know, as the word "Scharlachfieber" in German does not resemble "measles" at all, the latter being called "Masern" in my mother-tongue; but the thought that many a case, which had a bad issue, might have been treated, these twenty-one years, after my method, and many a life might have been saved, but for the mistake of C. C., has often distressed me.

[36] Nothing is more dangerous to the interest of an establishment, where many people are promiscuously collected, than a case of contagious disease, such as small-pox, scarlatina, measles, typhus, &c. I remember a hydriatic establishment in Pennsylvania being broken up entirely, and the physician deprived for a time of the means of subsistence, by his honest and well-founded confidence in the hydriatic treatment of small-pox, and by the generous steps he took in taking a friendless patient, afflicted with that dreaded disease, to his own house, to cure him. He anticipated the

pleasure it would procure him to show how quickly and how safely he would dispose of the case, and exulted in being able to communicate the fact to his patients. Alas, he little knew, how feeble their confidence in the water-cure was as yet, and how much more they thought of their own safety, than of the water-cure, their physician and the life and health of a poor destitute fellow-creature. They all left him — part of them came to Florence — and long before he had cured his small-pox patient, he had not one of his old patients left to witness the cure! However impolitic it may appear, I cannot but express my admiration of Dr. S.'s noble conduct on the occasion, who proved himself not only an honest adherer to our excellent mode of treatment, but also a kind and generous man, worthy of more encouragement than he received at the time.

With that event before me and with a number of some thirty-five or forty patients in the house, I, of course, tried to make them as easy as I could, and confiding in the power of my treatment, sent my own two children, *Paul*, about eight and a half, and *Eliza*, about four years old, to play with the little scarlet-patient, to show how little I was afraid of the disease. In doing so, I, at the same time, satisfied my own heart, by insuring the possibility of treating my darlings myself for scarlatina, which I might not be able to do, were I to let the opportunity escape. Both were taken by the disease, and finding their reaction rather torpid, and the whole process of the disease not without danger, I was glad — when all was over — that I had been able to treat them myself.

I am happy to declare, that none of *my* patients were frightened away, and that all those who were attacked by the contagion, came off in a very short time and without the least bad consequences. The only exception, in the case of a person who was not a patient, and who came under my hands, after other remedies had been tried on him, I shall communicate hereafter.

[Pg 80]

PART III.

113. TREATMENT OF OTHER ERUPTIVE FEVERS.

The treatment as prescribed for scarlatina in this pamphlet, is applicable also for other eruptive fevers, such as small-pox, varioloids, chicken-pocks, measles, miliaria, urticaria, zoster, rubeola, erysipelas, erythema, &c., its principal feature being the wet-sheet pack, which may always be safely employed, even by an inexperienced hand. It is not the object of this treatise to discuss all these different diseases in full: I shall do so in a larger work on the water-cure, which I intend to publish in English as soon as I find leisure enough to finish it. But I shall give, in the meanwhile, a few hints sufficient to guide the reader in their treatment.

114. SMALL-POX.

Small-pox, by far the most dangerous of them, has found a barrier in its destructive progress in Dr. Jenner's discovery. Vaccination is an almost sure prophylactic against it; but, notwithstanding, many, with whom the preservative was neglected or with whom it proved powerless, have fallen victims to its ravages. There is no remedy in the drug-stores to diminish the danger to which the life, health and appearance of those afflicted with this terrible disease are exposed. The only safe remedy is the wet-sheet pack.

The water for the sheet should be between sixty-five and seventy degrees, and the bath after the pack, from [Pg 81] 70 to 75°. Colder water is only applicable before the appearance of the eruption, which may be favored by frictions with bare hands dipped in it. These frictions may be repeated twice a day for the first two days. On the third day a long pack will call forth the eruption. If the patient can be kept in it, he may stay from three to five hours; adults even longer. No harm can be done by it, as the patient produces comparatively little heat, and the longer the pack the surer it will be to bring out the pocks. A short pack will have little effect.

As soon as the pocks appear, rubbing must be avoided till the scabs are entirely gone. The patient should be packed two, three, and even four times a day, according to the condition of the skin and the height of the fever. There is nothing able to relieve the patient as much as the dampness of the wet pack. During the period of eruption and efflorescence, the patient should spend the greater part of his time in the wet-sheet, which not only relieves the general symptoms, but especially the inflammation of the skin, and makes the poison less virulent, by constantly absorbing part of it, and by communicating part of its moisture to the small ulcers.

To protect the face, a kind of mask may be made of several thicknesses of linen, covering the whole of it, leaving openings only for the mouth, nostrils and eyes. The latter may be covered separately. This compress should be covered with one or two thicknesses of flannel, to keep its temperature as even as possible, for which purpose it should be changed as often as it becomes uncomfortably warm.

To draw the poison away from the face and eyes, it will be a good plan to put a thick wet compress on the back of the neck and between the shoulders, and cover it thickly, so as to create a great deal of heat in that region. It will bring out the pocks densely. It should be changed only when it becomes dry.

[Pg 82] The stomach should be covered also with a wet compress, as that organ is almost always in a bad state during the whole course of the disorder. If pus is received into the blood, the thick matter which is filtered through the kidneys frequently causes retention of urine. In that case the wet bandage should go around the body, and the patient should drink a good deal of water to attenuate the blood and the urine, and favor the discharge. In case of need, a sitz-bath of 75°—or with weak patients of a higher temperature, 80 to 90°—will remove the difficulty.

During convalescence, the baths should be made gradually colder, to invigorate the skin and the rest of the organism, and prepare the patient for going out, which may safely be permitted on the tenth or twelfth day. The packs ought to be continued for a week at least after the drying and falling off of the scabs.

By following this treatment, the patient will be safe from any bad consequences of the disease. I have never seen any of the usual sequelæ after packs.

115. VARIOLOIDS AND CHICKEN-POCKS.

Varioloids and *Chicken-pocks*, are treated in the same manner, but require less treatment. If well attended to, neither *small-pox*, nor *varioloids* or *chicken-pocks*, will leave any marks.

116. MEASLES.

Measles, which may be easily distinguished from scarlatina, by the symptoms I have given under 29, are to be treated like the mildest forms of scarlet-fever, and, in most cases, require no treatment at all. Nervous affections are treated like those of scarlet-fever (92, &c.). — As measles are more dangerous to adults than to children, whose skin is much more active, they had better take packs, without waiting for an increase of the symptoms.

[Pg 83] 117. URTICARIA, ZOSTER, RUBEOLA.

Urticaria, *Zoster* and *Rubeola*, are treated in the same manner as measles: the main feature, however, is the pack.

118. ERYSIPELAS.

Erysipelas being commonly the reflexion of an internal disease with a peculiar tendency towards the skin, should not be treated locally alone, but with due regard for the original disease. If possible, the patient should perspire freely in long packs, whilst a wet compress relieves the local inflammation. The compress, without the pack, would be apt to cause a metastasis to a vital organ. Sometimes a derivative compress, as mentioned under small-pox (114), will draw the inflammation away from a very painful and dangerous spot. It is advisable to try it, if the seat of the inflammation is the face or head. The water for the sheet, compress and bath should not be lower than 65°. I know several cases of rapid cures of erysipelas, by throwing a profusion of cold water on the parts affected. But, although I do not remember any harm done by such a process, I can scarcely recommend it, as long as there are milder and safer remedies at our disposal. [37]

119. ERYTHEMA.

Erythema may be considered an exceedingly mild form of erysipelas, and yields to gentle treatment, as it is given in measles.

120. ADDITIONAL RULES FOR THE TREATMENT OF ERUPTIVE DISEASES.

In all these eruptive diseases, especially small-pox, all I have said, in speaking of scarlatina, about ventilation, [Pg 84] air, diet, &c., ought to be duly observed. In small-pox, a constant renovation of the air is indispensable, as the morbid exhalations from the body of the patient are most offensive, and the contagious poison most virulent.

121. The temperature of the room, however, should be a few degrees higher than in scarlatina, as none of these other eruptive diseases shows the same degree of fever and heat. This is particularly advisable in the treatment of measles, when exposure is very apt to cause the rash to disappear, an occurrence which is dangerous in any eruptive disease.

122. CONCLUSIVE REMARKS. — OBSTACLES.

Before concluding my article, I shall attempt to remove a few objections and obstacles, which are usually raised against the practice of the hydriatic system in families.

123. WANT OF WATER.

One of the obstacles is the *want of a sufficient quantity of water* in some houses, and the difficulty of procuring it.

This obstacle is easily removed.

If you cannot procure water enough for a half-bath—for there cannot be a difficulty in procuring a pailful for wetting the sheet—give your patient a *dripping sheet* instead, which, in most cases, will do as well; or, should there be a want of a wash-tub to give it in, a *rubbing sheet* may supply the bath.

124. DRIPPING SHEET, SUBSTITUTE FOR THE HALF-BATH.

To apply the *dripping sheet*, a tin bathing hat or a large wash-tub is placed near the patient's bed, and a pail of water on the brim of the hat, or close by the tub. Dip a linen sheet into it, and leave it there till you wish to take the patient out of his pack, but dispose it so that you can easily find the two corresponding corners. As [Pg 85] soon as the patient steps into the hat or tub, seize the sheet by these corners and throw it over his head and body from behind, and rub him all over, head and all, whilst somebody else is supporting him, or whilst he is supporting himself by taking hold of one of the bedposts. When the sheet becomes warm, empty part of your pail over the patient's head, by which means the water in the sheet is renewed, and rub again. Then repeat the same operation, and when all your water is gone, before the body of the patient is sufficiently cool, take water from the hat or tub and use it for the same purpose, till he is quite cooled down. Then dry him with another sheet, or a towel, and put him to bed again, if necessary.

125. RUBBING SHEET, SUBSTITUTE FOR THE HALF-BATH.

It cannot be difficult to procure a wash-tub. Should you be so situated, however, as not to be able to procure even this, you will be compelled to make shift with a *rubbing sheet*. For that purpose, a sheet and a pail of water are all you need. The sheet is wetted in the pail and slightly wrung out. The patient steps on a piece of oil-cloth or carpet, and you throw your wet-sheet over him and rub, as before indicated. When the sheet is warm, you dip it in the pail again, and repeat the process, and thus you go on, till the patient is sufficiently cooled.

If you can have two pails of water, it will be better than one, as the water becomes warm after having changed the sheet a couple of times.

126. WHERE THERE IS A WILL, THERE IS A WAY!

I have been frequently compelled to resort to these milder applications, when there were no bathing utensils in families or boarding-houses, or no servants to carry the water for a bath; and they have always [Pg 86] answered very well. In cases where a sitz-bath or a half-bath is indispensable, to save the life of a patient, you will find the means of procuring bathing utensils and the necessary quantity of water.

Where there is a will, there is a way! — I am sure that when once your mind is made up to use the treatment, it will not be difficult for you to find the means for it. There is always water, and there are always hands enough, where there is *resolution*. And who would mind a little trouble, when he can save a fellow creature's, perhaps a darling child's life and health? As for the rest, the few days' trouble, which the hydriatic mode of treatment gives, is largely recompensed by the much shorter duration of the disease, and by the immediate relief the patient derives from almost every application of water.

I have generally found that those parents who had confidence in the treatment, had also the courage to resort to it. *Confidence and courage* create *resolution*, and when once you have begun to treat your patient, you will be sure to persevere. *Il n'y a que le premier pas qui coûte*, as the French say: only the first step is difficult.

127. PREJUDICE OF PHYSICIANS AGAINST THE WATER-CURE.

The greatest, and the most serious, difficulty lies in the prejudice of physicians against the Water-Cure. This prejudice, although in the treatment of the diseases before us, it is founded on no other reasons but ignorance, lack of courage and the habit of travelling the old trodden path—the same *regular path* which thousands and millions have travelled not to return—neither you, dear reader, nor I, shall be able to conquer by words. But we may succeed by actions. Take the matter in your own hands, before it is too late. Do not plead your want of knowledge and experience: a whip in the hand of a child is less dangerous than a double-edged sword in the [Pg 87] hand of a fencing-master. I have known many a mother to treat her child for scarlet-fever, measles, small-pox, croup, &c., after my books, or after prescriptions received in Græfenberg and other hydriatic establishments, and I scarcely remember a case of accident, whilst those treated in the usual mode by the best physicians would die in numbers. I repeat it: there is no danger in the *wet-sheet pack*, and should a patient die under the treatment prescribed by me, you may be sure, he would not have lived under any other mode of treatment.

128. REBELLION!

This is preaching rebellion!

I know it is, and it is with great reluctance that I preach it, as I am by no means in favor of taking medical matters out of the hands where they belong, to place them into the hands of such as have had no medical education. I despise quackery, and I wish physicians could be prevailed upon to take the matter in their own hands. But, the following anecdote will enable you to judge what we may expect in that quarter, and whether I am justified in preaching rebellion against the old routine—for I deny going against science and the profession—and for a new practice which has proved to be safer than any hitherto adopted.

129. FACTS.

In 1845-46 there was an epidemic in Dresden, a city of 100,000 inhabitants, where I then resided. Its ravages in the city and the densely peopled country around it, were dreadful. We had excellent physicians of different schools, who exerted themselves day and night to stop the progress of extermination, but all was in vain. Dying children and weeping mothers were found in some house of every street, and whenever you entered a dry-goods store, you were sure to find people buying [Pg 88] mourning. At last, as poverty will frequently produce dispute and quarrel in families, there arose, from similar reasons, a dispute between the different sects of physicians in the papers, which became more and more animated and venomous, without having any beneficial influence upon the dying patients. Sad with the result of the efforts, and disgusted with the quarrel of the profession, I gathered facts of my own and other hydriatic physicians' practice, by which it was shown that I alone, in upwards of one hundred cases of scarlatina, I had treated, had not lost a patient, and that, in general, not a case of death of scarlet-fever treated hydriatically was on record. These facts, with some observations about the merits of the respective modes of treatment, I published in the same papers, offering to give the list of the patients, I had treated, and to teach my treatment, gratis, to any physician who would give himself the trouble of calling.—What do you think was the result of my communication and offer?

The quarrel in the papers was stopped at once; not a line was published more; no one attempted to contradict me or to show that I had lost patients also; all was dead silence; and of the one hundred and fifty physicians of the city, *one* called, and, not finding me at home, never returned. And the patients? Well, the patients were treated and killed—after the occurrence I thought I had the right to use the word—as before, and the practice was continued in every epidemy afterwards.

Perhaps my communications would have had a better result in America, where physicians, though much less learned upon an average, are more accessible to new ideas? —

130. I have tried, several years ago, to have an article on the subject inserted in one or two of the New-York papers, which have the largest circulation in the country, [Pg 89] but, although there were at the time 150 deaths of scarlet-fever per week in the city, they had so much to say about slavery and temperance that there was no room for my article, and when I published it in the Water-Cure Journal, it was, of course, scarcely noticed. —Scarlet-patients have continued to be treated and to die as before, and when I published a couple of months ago an extract from this pamphlet in the Boston Medical World, there were thirty cases of death per week from scarlatina in that city.

These are facts, upon which you may make your own comments. But the following are facts also:

131. MORE FACTS!

I have been treating several hundred cases of eruptive fevers during twenty-one years, and except the one mentioned above (111.) never lost a patient. I have known similar results, in the practice of other hydriatic physicians who employed a similar method. I scarcely remember a bad result of hydriatic treatment undertaken by the parents and relations of the patient, without the assistance of any physician at all. I know of several cases of death, in scarlatina, where physicians attempted to employ Currie's method, without packing; [38] and I [Pg 90] have frequently seen the learning of regular physicians interfere with our simple practice and produce different results, whilst people without medical knowledge, by strictly adhering to my prescriptions, would always be successful. I have been so successful, and am so confident in the treatment, as described, that I have not only neglected to vaccinate my children (till last year, when it was done by a friend in my absence), but that I have sent them to a scarlet-patient to take the disease, in order that I might be able to treat them myself, and know them to be protected in future.

132. CONCLUSION: HELP YOURSELVES, IF YOUR PHYSICIANS WILL NOT HELP YOU!

And I am none of your water-enthusiasts, who pretend to cure everything and any thing with water. My confidence in the hydriatic treatment of eruptive fevers, however, is almost unlimited, because it is founded on an experience of many years of happy results with scarcely any exception, and on the fact that no other method can show a similar result.

I have always been considered an honest man, dear reader, and always anxious to serve my fellow-men; and what selfish view could I have in thus attempting to persuade you to save your children's lives by adopting my method of treatment? I shall neither make friends with the members of the profession by thus exciting you to rebel against the old routine, nor shall I augment the number of the patients of my establishment; for we cannot very well carry patients with scarlet-fever and small-pox to a distant institution. Believe me, I have no other object in publishing this pamphlet, than that of saving the life and health of as many human beings as possible, which otherwise would perish. In publishing this pamphlet, I intend to perform a sacred duty, without any regard to making a pleasant or unpleasant [Pg 91] impression upon my brother physicians, and consequently without any regard to my own interest.

The fact that I exposed my own youngest children, the pleasure, and the support *in spe*, of my declining age, to the contagion of scarlatina, during an epidemic which had rather a malignant character, proves more than any thing my honest confidence in my own remedy. Ask your physician, if he is adverse to the hydriatic method, whether he knows a remedy in which he has so much confidence as to be willing to imitate my example. There is no such remedy in the apothecary's shop, and there is no physician who would expose his own children to the contagion of scarlatina from the confidence he has in the curative or protective powers *of any drug*.

I hope, my brother-physicians will believe me, when I assure them, that I do not mean any disrespect to the profession, in thus introducing a new sound method for the weak old routine. Perhaps, my exposition of the principles of my practice, and the attempt at a systematic arrangement of the materials at my disposal, may gain a few converts. If I am not mistaken, this pamphlet is the first that treats the subject systematically and to some extent. I am aware that it might be better written and more perfect. But, I trust that it will do some good, and hope it will pave the way for a better production, based on a more extensive practice and enriched with new discoveries on the part of American physicians, whose genius and activity are not inferior to those of any other nation.

When the Hydriatic System becomes more and more a part of the practice of educated and enlightened practitioners, it will become a much greater benefit to the human race, not only with regard to the cure of eruptive fevers, but of that of all diseases to which it can be adapted, beside the happy reform it will assist in bringing about in our effeminate and luxurious way of living, [Pg 92] which, at all times, has been a source of ruin for individuals, families and nations.

But as long as the profession continues in its old routine, I can give you no other advice than that of following my prescriptions and of helping yourselves:—

"Aide-toi, et le ciel t'aidera!"

FOOTNOTES:

[37] I speak here of the true erysipelas, of course, and not of the chronic eruption of the face, &c., erroneously called erysipelas by many.

[38] I think of the obstinacy of a medical friend, who refused to take a lesson from Priessnitz, and constantly looked for advice, in cases of need, in works written by learned practitioners. He lost three patients in one family from scarlatina anginosa, which would certainly have been cured by the packs. In two other cases I was called to his assistance, when he insisted upon putting ice upon the head of the patients to remove the affection of the brain (the reaction was sthenic! See 50). I told him that in the cases before us, repeated packing was the only safe application, and we had a few unpleasant words, when I yielded, promising him that he would come round to my opinion within a few hours. And so it was; the

patients grew worse and worse, with their heads shaved and ice upon them, till my good friend requested me to take the rudder in my own hand, with the promise not to interfere any more. By packing, the patients improved visibly and were out of danger within two days.

CATALOGUE
[Pg 93] OF
HOMŒOPATHIC BOOKS,

FOR SALE BY
WILLIAM RADDE, 300 BROADWAY, NEW-YORK,
Between Duane and Reade-sts.,
(*late No. 822 Broadway,*)

PUBLISHER OF HOMŒOPATHIC BOOKS AND SOLE AGENT FOR THE LEIPZIG
CENTRAL HOMŒOPATHIC PHARMACY.

HOMŒOPATHIC MEDICINES.

Wm. Radde, 300 Broadway, New-York, respectfully informs the Homœopathic Physicians and the friends of the System, that he is the sole Agent for the Leipzig Central Homœopathic Pharmacy, and that he has always on hand a good assortment of the best Homœopathic Medicines, in complete sets or by single vials, in *Tinctures, Dilutions,* and *Triturations;* also *Pocket Cases of Medicines; Physicians' and Family Medicine Chests to Laurie's Domestic* (60 to 82 Remedies).—EPP'S (60 Remedies).—HERING'S (60 to 102 Remedies).—*Small Pocket Cases* at $3, with Family Guide and 27 Remedies.—Cases containing 415 Vials, with Tinctures and Triturations for Physicians.—Cases with 268 Vials of Tinctures and Triturations to Jahr's New Manual, or Symptomen-Codex.—Physicians' *Pocket Cases* with 60 Vials of Tinctures and Triturations.—Cases from 200 to 300 Vials, with low and high dilutions of medicated pellets.—Cases from 50 to 80 Vials of low and high dilutions, &c. &c. Homœopathic Chocolate. Refined Sugar of Milk, pure Globules, &c. *Arnica Tincture*, the best specific remedy for bruises, sprains, wounds, &c. *Arnica Plaster*, the best application for *Corns. Arnica salve, Urtica urens, tincture and salve*, and Dr. Reisig's *Homœopathic Pain Extractor* are the best specific remedies for *Burns. Canchilagua*, a Specific in Fever and Ague. Also Books, Pamphlets and Standard Works on the System in the English, French, Spanish and German Languages.

☞ Physicians ordering medicines will please mark after each one its strength and preparation as:

moth. tinct. for mother tincture.
1. *trit.* or 3. *trit.* for first or third trituration.
6. *in liq.* or 30 *in liq.* for sixth or thirtieth attenuation in liquid.
3. *in glob.* or 30 *in glob.* for third or thirtieth attenuation in globules.

Hartmann, Dr. F., Diseases of Children and their Homœopathic Treatment. Translated, with notes, and prepared for the use of the American and English Profession, by Charles J. Hempel, M. D. 1853. Bound, $2.00.

Jahr, Dr. G. H. G., The Homœopathic Treatment on the diseases of females. Translated from the French by Charles J. Hempel, M.D. large 8 vo. 1856. 422 Pages. Bound, $2.00.

Becker, Dr. A. C., On Constipation. Translated from the German, Bound, 38 cts.

Becker, Dr. A. C., On Consumption. Translated from the German, Bound. 38 cts.

Becker, Dr. A. C., On Dentition. Translated from the German, Bound, 38 cts.

Becker, Dr. A. C., On Diseases of the Eye. Translated from the German, Bound, 38 cts.

☞ The above four works by Dr. A. C. Becker, can be have bound in one volume, at $1.

Bryant, Dr. J., A Pocket Manual or Repertory of Homœopathic Medicines alphabetically and neologically arranged; which may be used as the physician's Vade-Mecum, the traveller's Medical Companion, or the Family Physician: containing the principal remedies for the most important diseases, symptoms, sensations, characteristics of diseases, &c.; with the principal pathogenetic effects of the medicines on the most important organs and functions of the [Pg 94] body; together with diagnosis, explanation of technical terms, directions for the selection and exhibition of remedies, rules of diet, &c., &c. Compiled from the best homœopathic authorities. Bound, $1.25.

Caspari's Homœopathic Domestic Physician, edited by F. Hartmann, M.D., "Author of the Acute and Chronic Diseases." Translated from the eighth German edition, and enriched by a Treatise on Anatomy and Physiology, embellished with 30 illustrations, by W. Esrey, M.D. With additions and a preface by C. Hering, M.D. Containing also a Chapter on Mesmerism and Magnetism; directions for patients living some distance from a homœopathic physician, to describe their symptoms; a Tabular Index of the medicines and the diseases in which they are used; and a Sketch of the Biography of Dr. Samuel Hahnemann, the Founder of Homœopathy. Bound $1.25.

Chepmell, Dr. E. C., Domestic Homœopathy restricted to its legitimate sphere of practice, together with rules for diet and regimen. First American edition, with additions and improvements by Samuel B. Barlow, M.D., Bound, 50 cts.

Curtis, J. T., M.D., and J. Lillie, M.D., Epitome of Homœopathic Practice. Compiled chiefly from Jahr, Rückert, Beauvais, Bœninghausen, &c. Second enlarged edition. Bound, 75 cts.

Douglas, Dr. J. S., Homœopathic Treatment of Intermittent Fevers. 1853, 38 cts.

Dudgeon's Lectures on the Theory and Practice of Homœopathy. Delivered at the Hahnemann Hospital School of Homœopathy, by R. E. Dudgeon, M.D. Manchester, 1854. Bound, (565 pages) $2.50.

Gollmann, Wm. M.D., The Homœopathic Guide, in all Diseases of the Urinary and Sexual Organs, including the derangements caused by Onanism and Sexual Excesses; and accompanied by an Appendix on the use of Electro-Magnetism in the Treatment of these diseases. Translated with Additions by Ch. J. Hempel. 1855. Bound, $1.50.

Guernsey, Dr. Egbert, The Gentleman's Hand-Book of Homœopathy; especially for travellers, and for Domestic Practice. 1855. Bound, 75 cts.

Hahnemann, Dr. Samuel, The lesser Writings of, collected and translated by R. E. Dudgeon, M.D. With a Preface and Notes by E. E. Marcy, M.D., With a beautiful steel engraving of Hahnemann, from the Statue by Steinhæuser. Bound, one large volume (784 pages). $3.00.

☞ This valuable work contains a large number of Essays of great interest to laymen as well as medical men, upon diet, the prevention of diseases, ventilation of dwellings, &c. As many of these papers were written before the discovery of the Homœopathic theory of cure, the reader will be enabled to peruse in this volume the ideas of a gigantic intellect when directed to subjects of general and practical interest.

"The Lesser Writings MUST BE READ by every student of Homœopathy who wishes to become acquainted with the *Master-mind.*" R. E. Dudgeon, M.D.

Hahnemann, Dr. Samuel, Materia Medica Pura. Translated by C. J. Hempel, M.D. 4 vols. Bound, $6.00.

Hahnemann, Dr. Samuel, The Chronic Diseases, their Specific Nature and Homœopathic Treatment. Translated and edited by C. J. Hempel, M.D., with a Preface by C. Hering, M.D., 5 vols. Bound, $7.00.

Hahnemann, Dr. Samuel, Organon of Homœopathic Medicine, third American edition, with Improvements and additions, from the last German edition, and Dr. C. Hering's introductory remarks. Bound, $4.00.

☞ The above four works of Dr. Samuel Hahnemann, are and will forever be the greatest treasures of Homœopathy; they are the most necessary works for Homœopathic Practitioners, and should grace the library of every Homœopathic Physician.

Hempel, Dr. **Charles Julius**, A Treatise on the use of Arnica, in cases of Contusions, Wounds, Sprains, Lacerations of the Solids, Concussions, Paralysis, Rheumatisms, Soreness of the Nipples, &c., &c., with a number of cases, illustrative of the use of that drug. 19 cts.

[Pg 95] **Hempel, Dr. Charles Julius**, Complete Repertory of the Homœopathic Materia Medica. 1224 pages. 1853. Bound, $6.00.

☞ We have now before us the result of Dr. Hempel's incessant labors in the shape of a portly volume of upwards of 1200 pages, for which he deserves the best thanks of the homœopathic body at large. This volume will be a great acquisition to all practitioners of our art, as it will facilitate very much their search for the appropriate remedy. — We have already made extensive use of it; thanking Dr. Hempel most heartily for his repertory, we commend it confidently to our English colleagues. It will be found useful by all, whether they possess the two volumes of the Symptomen-Codex or no; and, it will in many cases guide the practitioner to the ready discovery of an appropriate remedy, when all the other works hitherto published in our language would leave him in the lurch. — *From the British Journal of Homœopathy*, No XLIV.

I use it almost daily in my practice, and have frequently been able to find the symptom or group of symptoms wished for, in a few minutes on its pages, after having for a much longer time searched in vain through the older repertories.

Philadelphia **M. Williamson, M.D.**

I have ever found it reliable, and since becoming familiar with its arrangement, I regard it the best practical guide yet offered to the homœopathic profession in this country.

Philadelphia **A. E. Small, M.D.**

I consider it a work of merit and decidedly of use to Physicians commencing the practice of Homœopathy.

Philadelphia **James Kitchen, M.D.**, 215 Spruce-street.

Ever since your Repertory was issued, it has been my daily adviser, has never failed to assist me and has also saved me a great deal of time.

Philadelphia **Geo. Duhring, M.D.**

I place a high estimation upon the entire work, and shall consider it a safe guide to govern me in my prescriptions to the sick.

Philadelphia **Richard Gardiner, M.D.**

I can with truth say, that I consider it by very far the best Repertory I have ever used or seen, and that, I would by no means be without it. It has saved me many hours of research, and has very seldom failed to satisfy my expectations.

Philadelphia **J. R. Coxe, Jr. M.D.**

I deem it an act of justice to say that I believe it to be the best work of the kind in the English language,—and that it will be not only a valuable aid to the student, but greatly facilitate the practitioner of Homœopathy in the selection of remedies in the treatment of disease. The profession are under great obligation to Dr. Hempel for furnishing them with so valuable a work.

Philadelphia **Wm. Stiles, M.D.**

I have examined your new "Repertory" with much care, and I am happy to recommend it as a work eminently calculated to facilitate the labors of students as well as of practicing physicians in referring both to particular symptoms and the remedies calculated to meet those symptoms.

I believe it to be unequalled in this by any work of the kind published in America.

Philadelphia **M. Semple, M.D.** Prof. Chem. and Tox. Hom. Med. Col. Pa.

I have been requested to give my opinion of "Dr. Hempel's Repertory." It supplies, in my estimation, a desideratum, which entitles its author and publisher to the thanks of the whole Homœopathic school, and exhibits an amount of labor and research, which few men beside the indefatigable author would have been willing to undertake. I should consider no Homœopathic Library complete without it.

Philadelphia **Robt. T. Evans, Jr. M.D.**

I have frequently consulted the "Repertory of the Homœopathic Materia Medica," so ably compiled by Dr. Hempel, and do not hesitate to commend it to the attention of the adherents of Homœopathy.

New-York **A, Gerald Hull, M.D.**

Dr. Hempel's Repertory is an elaborate practical index to the Materia Medica and the only complete work of the kind in our language.

New-York **J. T. Curtis, M.D.**

I have used Hempel's Repertory almost from the first day of its publication, and I am more and more pleased with it, the more I use it. I make frequent reference to it, not only for assistance against the daily exigencies of medical practice, but in the composition of the medical work in which I have been for some time engaged, I am almost always sure to find the very information that I require. I have frequently quoted in my Treatises on Headache, Apoplexy, and Diseases of Females, and shall continue to quote in the forthcoming books.

The industry, and command of the English language possessed by Dr. Hempel, are truly wonderful.

New-York **J. C. Peters, M.D.**

Jahr's New Manual; originally published under the name of Symptomen Codex. (Digest of Symptoms.) This work is intended to facilitate a [Pg 96] comparison of the parallel symptoms of the various Homœopathic agents, thereby enabling the practitioner to discover the characteristic symptoms of each drug, and to determine with ease and correctness what remedy is most Homœopathic to the existing group of symptoms. Translated, with important and extensive additions from various sources, by Charles Julius Hempel, M.D., assisted by James M. Quinn, M.D., with revisions and clinical notes by John F. Gray, M.D.; contributions by Dr. A. Gerald Hull,

George W. Cook, and Dr. B. F. Joslin, of New-York; and Drs. C. Hering, J. Jeanes, C. Neidhard, W. Williamson, and J. Kitchen of Philadelphia; with a Preface by Constantine Hering, M.D., 2 vols., bound $14.00.

The third volume is issued as a separate work, under the title of *Complete Repertory* of the Homœopathic Materia Medica. By Charles J. Hempel, M.D. 1224 pages. Price $6, or all three volumes at $20.

Jahr's New Manual of Homœopathic Practice; edited, with Annotations, by A. Gerald Hull, M.D. From the last Paris edition. This is the fourth American edition of a very celebrated work, written in French by the eminent Homœopathic Professor Jahr, and it is considered the best practical compendium of this extraordinary science that has yet been composed. After a very judicious and instructive introduction, the work presents a Table of the Homœopathic Medicines, with their names in Latin, English and German; the order in which they are to be studied, with their most important distinctions and clinical illustrations of their symptoms and effects upon the various organs and functions of the human system. The second volume embraces an elaborate of Analysis of the indications in disease, of the medicine adapted to cure, and a Glossary of the technics used in the work, arranged so luminously as to form an admirable guide to every medical student. The whole system is here displayed with a modesty of pretension, and a scrupulosity in statement, well calculated to bespeak candid investigation. This laborious work is indispensable to the students and practitioners of Homœopathy, and highly interesting to medical and scientific men of all classes. Complete Symptomatology and Repertory, 2 vols., bound, $6.00.

Jahr's, Dr. **G. H. G.** and **Possart's** New Manual of the Homœopathic Materia Medica, arranged with reference to well authenticated observations at the sick-bed, and accompanied by an alphabetical Repertory, to facilitate and secure the selection of a suitable remedy in any given case. 4th edition, enlarged by the Author. Symptomatology and Repertory. Translated and edited by C. J. Hempel, M.D. Bound, $3.50.

Joslin, Dr. **B. F.**, Principles of Homœopathia, In a series of lectures. Bound, 75 cts.

Joslin, Dr. **B. F.**, Homœopathic Treatment of Cholera including Repertories for this disease and for Summer-Complaints. Third edition with Additions. 1854. Bound, $1.

Homœopathic Cookery. Second edition, with additions, by the Lady of an American Homœopathic Physician. Designed chiefly for the use of such persons as are under Homœopathic treatment. 50 cts.

Laurie, Dr. J., The Parent's Guide. Containing the Diseases of Infancy and Childhood and their Homœopathic Treatment. To which is added a Treatise on the Method of rearing Children from their earliest Infancy; comprising the essential branches of Moral and Physical Education. Edited, with Additions by Walter Williamson, M.D., Professor of Matera Medica and Therapeutics in the Homœopathic Medical College of Pennsylvania (460 pages.) 1854. Bound, $1.00.

Laurie's Homœopathic Domestic Medicine. Arranged as a practical work for Students. Containing the treatment of Diseases and a Glossary of medical terms. Sixth American edition, enlarged and improved, by A. Gerald Hull, M.D. 1853. With full description of the dose to each single case. (800 pages.) Fourteenth thousand. Bound, $1.50.

www.ingramcontent.com/pod-product-compliance
Lightning Source LLC
Chambersburg PA
CBHW030442220526
45464CB00006B/2377